Unmasking Acne: The Definitive Guide to Clear Skin

Why Acne Products Don't Work and How You Can Get Permanently Clear Skin from Within

By: Sam Wood

Copyright 2021 by GoodGlow.co

All rights reserved. This book or any portion thereof may not be preproduced in any manner whatsoever without the written permission of the publisher except for the use of brief quotations or in a book review.

1st Edition, 2021

info@goodglow.co

https://goodglow.co

Table of Contents

Disclaimer iv

Introduction: What this Book is *Not* 1

Section I: The Acne Myth 5

Chapter 1: Acne, a Modern Disease 6

Chapter 2: The Real Root Causes of Acne 10

Chapter 3: Why Acne Products Don't Work 31

Section II: Diet 40

Chapter 4: Myths, Misconceptions and Mistakes 41

Chapter 5: Foods That Trigger Acne's Root Causes........46

Chapter 6: Clear Skin Food List 66

Chapter 7: How to Analyze Any Food for Clear Skin ...122

Section III: Meal Timing & Fasting 128

Chapter 8: Intermittent Fasting for Clear Skin 131

Chapter 9: Prolonged Fasting for Clear Skin 137

Chapter 10: Fasting for Clear Skin Best Practices 142

Section IV – Lifestyle & Supplements 149

Chapter 11: Supplements for Clear Skin 151

Chapter 12: Sleep, Stress, and Exercise 163

Chapter 13: Natural Skincare 169

Section V: Protocols 176

Chapter 14: Clear Skin Diet Blueprint Protocol.............179

Chapter 15: Insulin Reduction Protocol 197

Chapter 16: Gut Protocol 207

Chapter 17: Bacterial/Yeast Overgrowth Protocol.........215

Chapter 18: Fungal Acne Protocol 220

Chapter 19: Carnivore Protocol......................................232

Chapter 20: Plant-Based Protocol 240

Chapter 21: Thyroid Protocol...248

Closing Thoughts 255

Resources to Use *Right Now* 257

About the Author...258

Bibliography..259

Disclaimer

The author of this book is not a doctor, physician assistant, nurse practitioner, nurse, or in the health profession. Information in this book cannot be used to diagnose, cure, or treat any disease. Do not follow any recommendations in this book without first discussing it with your medical professional. All content found within this book or on the GoodGlow website, including text, images, audio, or other formats, were created for informational purposes only. The content is not intended to be a substitute for professional medical advice, diagnosis, or treatment. Always seek the advice of your physician or other qualified health provider with any questions you may have regarding a medical condition. Never disregard professional medical advice or delay in seeking it because of something you have read in this book.

In everyday, plain English: I am *not* a doctor, registered dietician, nutritionist, or healthcare professional. I'm simply someone who has been interested in the scientific link between acne and underlying internal factors, like diet and inflammation, and who has seen success in treating acne with subsequent diet and lifestyle adjustments. This is *not* a substitute for medical advice in any way, shape, or form. This is for informational purposes only.

Introduction: What this Book is *Not*

I'm truly excited that you've decided to begin the journey towards achieving clear skin from within. I also want to congratulate you as you've already achieved one of the most important steps – making the *decision* to take control of your health and your skin. Traveling down this path was the single best decision for my health, self-esteem, and overall wellbeing that I ever made, and I hope it will be for you too.

Still, while this is all very exciting, I think that it's important to clear up what this book is *not*. This book takes an unconventional approach to beating acne, because, well, acne is an unconventional disease. As you'll learn shortly, acne, while appearing on the surface of the skin, is really a disease that begins *underneath* the skin, with hormones, inflammation, the gut microbiome, and a whole lot more. That's why this book will *not* be covering topical products (creams, ointment, gels, etc.) or cleaning regimens in extreme detail.

The reason for this is simple: acne is primarily an *internal* disease, and treating it topically, even if those topical products are "natural," is only covering up the *symptoms* of acne, not treating the *root causes*. There will be a brief section in the Lifestyle & Supplements section on natural skincare, as well as a scientific explanation as to why *most* acne products only make acne worse, in both the Root Causes section and several other chapters throughout the book. Our primary focus will be improving our *internal* health so that our skin can look great.

I know this may sound a bit overwhelming, but this book is designed to give *digestible* and *actionable* information to help you achieve your skincare goals. You can do this.

The Most Important Lesson I've Learned

If I can offer one word of wisdom before beginning this book, it's this: don't worry, we're going to get through this together.

I don't want to sound dramatic, but deciding to take control of my skin by changing my diet and lifestyle was the best decision I ever made. Still, one regret I have is how stressed out and obsessive I was at the beginning of the process, due to unrealistic expectations. I would spend insane amounts of time trying to find natural topical alternatives to acne medications that never seemed to work. I was tracking all the foods I was eating to make sure that everything matched up perfectly and stressed out about eating only the highest-quality, organic fruits and vegetables.

In the end, all of the obsessing over little things only made things worse, or at least slowed down my healing. This book isn't about getting everything *just right*. There will be flare-ups, there will be setbacks, and there will be challenges, but my goal is to help you cultivate a lifestyle that is *truly* proactive so that you don't have to worry about topical skincare or diet-driven flareups ever again. More importantly, I want you to be able to do this in a comfortable, caring way.

I'll be the first one to tell you that your skin isn't going to miraculously heal overnight. It might take weeks or months to show results, and if you beat yourself up during that time, you're only going to make it harder on yourself. You're likely going to have to make some challenging changes and do some challenging things. These aren't easy, but they're worth it, and at your own pace we'll get through this together. By the end of this process, your beautiful, radiant skin will be a side-effect of your own health, and you need to trust that real, lasting change doesn't come without resistance and hardships.

This book is a *guide*. A roadmap. It's not the law. It's not a rigid diet that you need to follow or a precise plan that you have to adhere to. If it helps you to treat it that way, then by all means, go for it! But throughout this book, you'll find areas where I encourage you to find what works for *you*. There is no one-size-fits all plan for acne – we all have different guts, different bodies, and different minds.

You can do this, and I'll help guide you along the way.

How To Read This Book

This book is broken down into several sections, each with its own special purpose for giving you the tools you need to beat acne for good. While you're welcome to skip around, I highly recommend reading each section so that you have a solid understanding of not only *what* you should eat or shouldn't eat for clear skin, but also *why*.

The simple fact of the matter is that everyone's body is different, and everyone reacts differently to different foods, supplements, and strategies. If you only understand what you should or shouldn't eat without understanding the reasoning behind it, you might stumble upon a diet plan that works well for other people but doesn't work for you, or you might find that a supplement that's supposed to help get rid of acne isn't doing the trick.

All the strategies discussed in this book are going to vary fin effectiveness rom individual to individual. By reading each section completely, you'll arm yourself with the tools necessary to make your own decisions and figure out a plan that works for *you*.

This book will be divided into 5 main parts, each with the goal of allowing you to fight acne from within and win:

1. **The Acne Myth:** Learn the *Real* Root Causes of Acne
2. **Clear Skin Diet:** A Comprehensive Overview of the Safest and Most Dangerous Foods for Acne
3. **Meal Timing for Clear Skin:** Intermittent and Prolonged Fasting for Clear Skin
4. **Lifestyle & Supplements:** How to Supercharge Your Diet and Beat Acne Fast
5. **Protocols:** Specific, Actionable Acne-Fighting Plans for Wherever You Are in Your Journey

By the end of this book, no matter where you currently are with your diet or what you've tried in the past, you'll have the tools you need to succeed.

But to begin with, we need to start with the basics – how, and more importantly *why,* does acne form in the first place? Why do certain cultures show no signs of acne, even in adolescents, while it seems like *everyone* in America and Europe struggle with acne? If we understand this, we can start our journey towards clear skin from within.

Section I: The Acne Myth

Chapter 1: Acne, a Modern Disease

If you're like me, you were told when you were young that acne was primarily caused by poor hygiene, dirty skin, or genetics. While there's a bit of truth to the genetics part, the fact of the matter is simple – acne is largely a disease caused by underlying, *internal* health conditions. If you're reading this book, you probably already had a hunch that this was somewhat true.

Despite the hundreds and possibly even thousands of dollars I spent on skincare products, and the hours upon hours of meticulous dedication to my skincare routine, I kept getting acne. Sometimes a new product would seem to work for a few weeks, only for me to have my acne coming back stronger than ever afterwards. I tried antibiotics, retinols, and just about every cleanser, cream, and contraption under the sun to try and get rid of it. I could cover up the symptoms of acne, but I never seemed to be able to get to the *root* cause.

If this sounds familiar, you're not alone – the acne industry alone generates 3 billion dollars of revenue a year[1], and rates of acne in first-world countries are at all-time highs. We have instant access to more miracle products than ever before, yet more and more of us have acne.

The underlying reason why acne products don't work is the same reason I wrote this book: topical acne products don't treat the *root causes* of acne; they only treat the symptoms. Acne is, primarily, an internal condition, a disease from *within* the body, and the evidence for this claim is growing year after year. We'll go over dozens of studies throughout this book, but just to whet your appetite, here are a few of the most striking: one study found that a diet which avoided insulin-spiking refined carbohydrates healed acne at twice the rate of the control diet. Another found that simply by taking a zinc supplement over the course of 12 weeks, patients saw a 50% decrease in acne.

Yet dermatologists to this day stand by the fact that diet has *nothing*, or at least very little, to do with acne (probably because if they *did* acknowledge this very simple fact, they'd be out of a job).

Perhaps the most provocative study around acne was one done by researcher Loren Cordain, who showed that rates of acne in the South American Aché tribe were a staggering zero[2]. That's right, ZERO. Even though the Ache Tribe's youth went through all the hormonal changes of adolescence, including fluctuating testosterone and estrogen, *none* of them had acne. It was the same story with the adults – not a sign of acne in sight.

Meanwhile, rates of acne in western societies are higher than ever. It's not surprising that upwards of 90% of adolescents have acne, but what's shocking is that 54% of women and 40% of men *older than 25 have acne*[2]. The skincare industry wants us to think of acne as something that comes and goes with puberty, but the simple fact of the matter is that *most* of us won't grow out of our acne, at least not anytime soon. So if you have acne and it doesn't seem to go away no matter what you do, you're not alone, not by a long shot.

What's the difference between the acne-free Aché and your typical American (or Brit, or Canadian, for that matter)? How could the Aché achieve perfectly clear skin without the acne cleansers, miracle creams, and antibiotics that seem to flood the current skincare market? In a single word – their *diet*.

Sure, the Aché are probably more active, in the sun more and less sedentary, but *by far* the largest difference between the Aché and the average person is in what they eat, and when. The Aché diet is heavy in meat, palm starch, honey, and some fruits. I don't want to focus too much on these particular foods, because what's important isn't the exact foods that the Aché eat, but rather what they *don't* eat. You won't find any processed foods, added sugars, or fried delicacies in the Aché diet which are so commonplace in western diets. The same goes for other hunter-gatherer tribes and native groups, like the Kitavan, Sapara, and Achur with astoundingly low rates of acne – they have diets low in processed foods and high in whole-food plants and animals.

Evolutionarily, this makes sense – our body has evolved over an extremely long period of time and refined carbohydrates like bread, or seed oils like canola oil, are relatively new inventions in the world of food. Meat, seafood, vegetables, fruit, nuts, seeds, and roots, on the other hand, have been consumed for tens of thousands of years, albeit in very different varieties than what we do today. Your body knows *exactly* how to digest blackberries because it's been molded by natural selection to do so over millennia. The damaging plant-proteins found in bread, on the other hand, are new, invasive, and challenging for your body to digest, which, as we'll talk about in the next chapter, leads to acne.

Now I'm not here to idolize our "hunter-gatherer" roots or claim that you need to give up all the conveniences of modern society in order to get clear skin. I'm simply referencing these studies because we finally are beginning to gather the evidence necessary to start tying together a cohesive story about the *real* root causes of acne – and this story seems to point in the direction of diet, nutrition, lifestyle, and stress.

It's got to the point now where to deny the evidence that acne is influenced by dietary and lifestyle factors is simply preposterous. *Thousands* of individuals have shared their stories with me about how cutting out a particular food, taking a certain supplement, or altering their meal timing led to a profound shift in their skin that acne products could never reproduce.

Still, you don't need to look any further than your own experience with acne to know that this is at least partially true. Ask yourself the following questions:

If you're eating well, exercising a lot, and generally taking care of your physical and mental health, do you find your skin to be a bit clearer?

Have you ever tried a product that seems to work for a while but which then ends up making your acne worse?

How many products have you tried over the years to try and get clear skin? Why have none of them worked?

Acne, as we'll explore in the next chapter, is an *internal* disease, and this book is going to teach you the *evidence-based* foundations necessary to get permanently clear skin from within. You won't have to worry about the acne cycle anymore and wondering what you can put on your skin and what you can't. No more complicated routines and hundreds of dollars down the drain.

But before we get there, we need to make a quick detour so that we can better understand *what* acne is, and more importantly, *why* we get acne. Once we understand these two points, we can start to develop a strategy to prevent acne. If you're still skeptical, read on. Analyzing these root causes and understanding the basic biology behind acne will make it abundantly clear that acne, while appearing on the surface of the skin, really forms and begins as an internal process.

Chapter 2: The Real Root Causes of Acne

Acne vulgaris, or acne for short, is a disease that affects the skin, typically on the face, but also on the back, chest, neck, or arms. At its core, acne is a bacterial infection followed by an inflammatory response from the body. The process of acne forming is relatively straightforward:

1. The body produces excess skin cells and/or sebum oil
2. Dead skin cells and/or sebum oil clog the pore
3. Acne bacteria swarm the clogged pore and infect it
4. The body triggers an inflammatory response - creating a big, protruding, red pimple

For now, this simple process is all you need to understand about acne – pores get clogged, infection occurs, and inflammation takes over. What's important *isn't* the scientific lingo around *how* acne forms, but rather *why* this process occurs in the first place:

- Why does our body produce too many skin cells or too much sebum oil?
- Why do pores get clogged in the first place?
- Why do big, red, protruding inflammatory comedones (also known as pimples) form?

And, most importantly, why do acne products not prevent these things from happening in the long run? The answers to these questions are the *root causes* of acne.

Overview: The 3 *Main* Root Causes of Acne

While there are hundreds, possibly of thousands of biological mechanisms that *can* contribute to acne (far too many to list here), our current clinical research points to three main root causes playing a role in just about every type of acne: insulin (hormones), inflammation, and indigestion.

Root Cause #1: Insulin and Other Acne-Causing Hormones

When we think of "hormonal acne," we usually think that sex hormones like testosterone and estrogen are the culprit. While this is partially true, it paints an incomplete picture of hormonal acne, and it makes us believe that acne is something that just comes up during puberty when levels of sex hormones increase, and that the acne will leave after these hormones are done.

DHT and estrogen, sex hormones found in both men and women that rise during puberty, *can* cause the skin to produce excess oil, which *can* lead to clogged pores and acne, but this isn't *necessarily* the case. More than half the individuals with acne during puberty *continue* to have acne after puberty, and many people don't even start developing acne until adulthood[1]. Even after sex hormone levels have died down, we still find ourselves with acne. Furthermore, despite rates of acne being higher than ever before, testosterone levels are actually *lower* than they were in previous decades[3].

Plus, remember the Aché tribe with a zero percent rate of acne that I mentioned earlier? Their adolescents undoubtably go through the hormonal transitions of puberty, yet *none* of them had acne. Sex hormones *can* contribute, or worsen, acne, but you won't *necessarily* have acne if you have high levels of sex hormones.

The reason for this is simple – sex hormones aren't the only hormones that cause acne, and in fact, there is a hormone that has an even larger effect on acne than DHT and estrogen – insulin.

Insulin 101

Insulin is a hormone secreted by the pancreas that helps break down the carbohydrates found in food into *usable* energy for the body. Basically, after you eat something, a form of sugar called glucose enters the bloodstream (blood sugar). Glucose in the bloodstream isn't really an ideal energy source for the body – it can't be used by muscles or tissues, which need something called *glycogen* to function.

You can think of the body like a car. Glucose is like raw oil before it's processed into gasoline. Cars need gasoline, and our body needs glycogen, so glucose won't do the trick, but we can turn glucose into *usable* energy with a little bit of help – that help comes from insulin.

To aid in storing and using this energy, the pancreas releases insulin, a hormone that travels through the body and helps cells convert and absorb the glucose found in the blood. Some of the glucose is used by the cells, and some of it is stored as *glycogen* (fuel) for later.

For some of us, this process works just fine – the body releases enough insulin to fulfill its needs, but not too much or too little. Insulin by itself isn't evil – it's only when we have *too much insulin* that we begin to get into problems related to acne. This is a condition called insulin resistance, and it affects upwards of half the American population[4]. Furthermore, it's a *huge* factor in hormonal acne. Insulin resistance might seem complicated, but it's a pretty simple process.

Imagine that you're packing a suitcase. You finish putting all your clothes in, and now it's time to put your shoes in. There's still a bit of room left, so it's not a huge deal - you'll just jam in the shoes and close the suitcase. Oops! You forgot that you also need to pack a suit. You manage to squeeze everything in and now you are barely able to even zip the suitcase shut. Shoot! You forgot you need to pack a beach towel, too! At this point, unless you take something out of the suitcase, it seems unlikely you're going to be able to even close it without throwing out your back.

I know it sounds like a silly analogy, but your body is a bit like this suitcase, and glucose in the bloodstream is like the extra shoes or towel that you're trying to fit in. When you eat food, the glucose is converted to glycogen and stored in the body for future use. But when you consistently eat more carbs (or foods that spike blood sugar levels, like dairy) than you need, it becomes harder and harder to "pack" more energy into the body, because all your cells are already full of usable glycogen. To force the blood sugar into the cells, you release more and more insulin to get the same job done. Unless you *use* some of the energy (by exercising, walking, etc.), it's going to be really hard for the body to pack all that glucose into the body. Repeat this cycle over and over again, and you have insulin resistance – a condition where the body releases way too much insulin anytime you eat certain foods.

Insulin and Acne

Insulin resistance is problematic for several different reasons – it's associated with a higher risk of certain diseases, can lead to chronic fatigue, and if you're not careful, will lead to diabetes (insulin resistance is oftentimes called prediabetes for this reason). But what we're worried about for now is how insulin causes acne.

The most important thing to remember is that insulin doesn't act alone – when your body produces insulin, it also produces a series of other hormones and molecules throughout the body.

Many of these insulin-triggered hormones and molecules are behind the root causes of acne. There are three that we're going to focus on here – Insulin-like Growth Factor 1 (IGF-1), Interleukin 1 Alpha (IL-1 Alpha), and Insulin-Like Growth Factor Binding Protein 3 (IGFBP-3).

I know these names probably sound complicated, but there's no need to worry about the specifics of each. We'll quickly go over how each contributes to acne, but the important thing to remember is that *insulin* is the single largest trigger for these three other acne-causing hormones and compounds.

Acne-Causing Hormone #1: IGF-1

IGF-1 is one of the single most important hormones to look at when it comes to acne. One of IGF-1's primary roles is letting your body know how many new cells to create. It's a growth hormone – it regulates the rate at which the body creates new cells and replaces old ones. IGF-1 is great if you're looking to bulk up, gain muscle mass, or recover faster from workouts, but for your skin, high levels of IGF-1 is generally a bad thing.

Because IGF-1 is a growth hormone, it triggers your body to produce a *ton* of new skin cells. These skin cells are created far beneath the surface of the skin and slowly rise up over a period of roughly 30 days. When this big batch of skin cells reach the surface of the skin, they compete for space and resources and end up actually blocking the pore. This blocked pore is the perfect breeding ground for infection and inflammation to take hold and for acne to form.

On top of that, IGF-1 also triggers other hormones that tell our skin to produce more sebum oil. Sebum oil can easily become oxidized (damaged) and clog pores. Worse yet, IGF-1 actually decreases our ability to handle oxidative stress. When oil on the skin becomes damaged or infected, we need *anti*oxidants to prevent further oxidation and damage from occurring, and IGF-1 *decreases* our body's ability to fight this oxidation. So not only does IGF-1 trigger more skin oil to be produced, but it also hinders our ability to prevent this oil from becoming oxidized, blocking pores and causing acne. It's no surprise that researchers have found a strong link between IGF-1 and acne[5].

Just like insulin, the key to IGF-1 is balance. You need some IGF-1 to properly function, grow, and repair, but not too much so you're producing tons of unnecessary skin cells. The problem in today's world is that consuming tons of carbs and dairy is the norm, so we're constantly producing way too much IGF-1 for our own good.

Acne-Causing Hormone #2: IGFBP-3

IGFBP-3 controls how quickly your skin cells die off and get replaced. High levels of IGFBP-3 causes skin cells to stick to each other and form rough scales on the surface of the skin. These scales then end up blocking the pore from the outside air, making it prone to infection and inflammation.

Combine IGFBP-3 and IGF-1 and you get a pretty nasty combination: too many skin cells are being produced, they stick to each other on the surface of the skin, and they're not being shed fast enough. The end result is that you have a ton of dead, rough, scaly skin cells that can easily clog pores.

Acne-Causing Compound #3: IL-1 Alpha

IL-1 alpha is what's called cytokine, which basically means that it's a small compound that acts as a "signal". IL-1 alpha signals an inflammatory response to the body, so that when the pore does become blocked and infected from IGF-1 and IGFBP-3,

IL-1 helps turn it into an inflamed, red, angry pimple. In many cases, this increased inflammation is the only thing that makes an underlying acne infection visible on the surface of the skin.

Summary: Insulin-Driven Acne

Remember the process we outlined earlier on how acne forms?

1. A pore becomes blocked or clogged by excess skin cells or sebum oil
2. An infection takes place
3. An inflammatory response is triggered

Well, these insulin-like hormones are all *directly* related to the physiological process of acne forming on the surface of the skin:

1. IGF-1 and IGFBP-3 blocks pores
2. IGF-1 increases oil production
3. IL-1 and IGF-1 promotes inflammation

As you can see, insulin, and the hormones that accompany insulin, contribute to all three of the root causes of acne, which is why there is no surprise that one study found that fasting insulin levels (a good marker of insulin resistance) were over 50% higher in patients with severe acne when compared to individuals without acne[6]. Combined with the fact that more than half of all Americans are considered "prediabetic" (in other words, they have insulin resistance), you can easily see why this is a problem for acne.

Still, like I said, insulin isn't evil – the key is making sure you have a healthy insulin response, and if necessary, decreasing your intake of foods that produce this hormone. In the next section, we're going to go over, in detail, the foods that trigger the most insulin and tactics that you can use to prevent insulin resistance from occurring, but for now let's move on to the next root cause of acne – inflammation.

Root Cause #2: Inflammation

Inflammation, just like insulin, isn't inherently bad. Basically, inflammation is our body's basic mechanism to help heal and protect the body. It's our natural response to foreign invaders, like toxins, bacteria, viruses, and physical damage. In moderation, inflammation is a good thing. When you get a cut or bruise, inflammation is your body's way of making sure it doesn't get infected. You wouldn't survive if it wasn't for inflammation. Inflammation only becomes problematic when it becomes *chronic*, or, in other words, when we have an overactive immune system that triggers inflammatory events too often.

Unfortunately, just like insulin, inflammation and chronic inflammation are more common than ever before. They can be triggered by extremely common ingredients found in everyday foods – even "healthy" foods, like yogurt, protein bars, and salad dressings. It's no surprise that rates of both chronic inflammation and acne are at all-time highs[7].

With chronic inflammation, your immune system (which responds to threats like viruses, bacteria, and other foreign invaders) is overly active. It treats everything like a major threat, even if it really isn't dangerous. Stress, naturally occurring infections, and even certain foods become sources of inflammation. These are routine bodily functions, but because of an overactive immune system, your body responds to them like serious threats – one of these "routine bodily functions" is, you guessed it, acne infections.

An acne infection isn't all that dangerous or threatening to the body. It doesn't take a large inflammatory response to make sure no damage is done, but when you suffer from chronic inflammation, your body thinks any infection is a huge threat. Even small acne infections caused by a blocked pore put your immune system on high alert. Tons of pro-inflammatory cells called cytokines are sent to the pore to clean up the mess. In order to stop this harmless acne infection, your body responds as if it were a serious cut or injury – by producing a red, protruding, inflamed comedo, or pimple.

In summary, acne *is* an inflammatory response – pimples are the byproduct of inflammation in response to a bacterial infection. This is yet another reason why using harsh chemicals or cleansers won't get rid of most acne – chronic inflammation is an immune response which occurs inside the body, not on the surface of the skin. While some anti-inflammatory topicals can help with the appearance of acne, they're only treating the surface level issue of inflammation.

That's why it's crucial to tackle acne at the source: by fixing the dietary imbalances and triggers that lead to chronic inflammation.

How Our Consumption of Unhealthy Fats Cause Chronic Inflammation

Just like the other root causes of acne, chronic inflammation is largely a side-effect of our modern diet and lifestyle. The main culprit: our increased consumption of unhealthy, industrialized fats.

Note: Digestive issues and food intolerances are also a major cause of both inflammation and insulin, which is why I consider them to be their own root cause – for this reason, they will be covered in the next section. All the root causes connect with each other and influence one another.

Before we even get into this topic, I need to start out by saying that fat is *not* evil. In fact, many fats are extremely healthy for you and your skin. I actually recommend that most individuals struggling with insulin and inflammation-related acne start out by *decreasing* carb consumption and *increasing healthy* fat consumption (again, we'll cover this in the next section).

The problem isn't fat in general, but a specific type of fats that are inflammatory, known as polyunsaturated omega-6 fatty acids. For years the USDA told us that in order to be healthy, we needed to avoid healthy, saturated fats and instead eat plenty of whole grains and refined carbohydrates. The end result is that both consumers and food producers alike have replaced these healthy fats (like coconut oil, extra-virgin olive oil, and ghee butter) with unhealthy, acne-causing industrial fats (like vegetable oils and margarine).

The reason for this is pretty straightforward – these seemingly healthy fats look a lot better on a nutrition label. If you believe that "saturated fat is evil," then these processed, low-saturated-fat vegetable oils, like canola, corn, or sunflower oil, *seem* like they're a lot better for you than saturated fats like coconut or olive oil. In reality, the exact opposite is true. It's not *saturated* fat we need to worry about, but *polyunsaturated* fat.

Polyunsaturated Fats, Omega-3, Omega-6, and Inflammatory Acne

In the world of fats, none are more important for how our body handles inflammatory responses than polyunsaturated fats, and more specifically, two *types* of polyunsaturated fats – Omega-3 and Omega-6:

- Omega-3 Fats: Anti-inflammatory. More Omega-3s means less inflammation, which means less acne

- Omega-6 Fats: Pro-inflammatory. More Omega-6s means more inflammation, which means more acne

Your body needs both fats to thrive. Omega-6 isn't completely evil – it's necessary for brain development, hair growth, and a well-functioning immune system, it's just that too much omega-6 can lead to chronic inflammation. Basically, you need to balance the amount of omega-6 fatty acids you eat with omega-3 fatty acids, otherwise you're likely to trigger large inflammatory responses.

Before humans started consuming vegetable and seed oils, it's estimated that our omega ratio, or the amount of omega-6 fats we consumed versus the amount of omega-3 fats, was somewhere around 1:1, meaning we ate equal amounts of omega-3s and omega-6s. Some estimates say it was closer to 2:1, meaning we ate 2x as many omega-6s. For clear skin, an omega ratio of somewhere between 2:1 and 4:1 is ideal, meaning you want to consume no more than 2-4x as much omega-6 as you do omega-3.

Now, given that information, where would you guess your omega ratio is at?

If you're like most Americans, you probably eat a shocking 10 times more omega-6 fatty acids than omega-3 fatty acids[8], which can lead to an increased risk of cardiovascular disease, cancer, and autoimmune disorders[9] (which is particularly important for acne). When your omegas are out of balance your immune system is constantly on high alert, and the likelihood that your body will produce an inflammatory response to an acne infection is greatly increased.

In the next chapter, we'll go over exactly which foods are highest in omega-6 fatty acids (and which foods are highest in omega-3 fatty acids, which are great for your skin), but for now, it's important to realize that, just like with insulin, most of us have diets which contain foods loaded with omega-6 fatty acids, *even if you're eating "healthy" foods.* Unless you have already gone out of your way to eliminate all vegetable oils from your diet, you're probably pumping your body full of inflammation-causing fats without even knowing it.

The important thing to remember for now is this: acne is an inflammatory disease – even if an acne infection occurs on the skin, which it often does, inflammation is what makes that simple little infection a visible, bright, red, pimple or blackhead.

Root Cause #3: Intolerances and Other Digestive Issues

High consumptions of omega-6 or insulin aren't the only culprits for inflammation-driven acne – food intolerances, reactions to certain antinutrients found in many foods, and other digestive issues also play major roles in acne – in fact, this specific type of inflammation is so important that we're going to treat it as its own root cause under the label of "Intolerances and Digestive Issues".

It has different triggers than other types of inflammation, and understanding this type of inflammation is absolutely crucial for beating acne from within – in fact, I would actually argue that it's the *most* important, simply because each and every person will have different intolerances and digestive issues that they bring to the table. If we can understand why and where our digestive system is triggering acne-causing inflammation, we can start to beat it from within.

Digestive Issue #1: Intestinal Permeability

The first major type of digestive issue that affects people with acne is oftentimes called "leaky gut syndrome."

Note: There is major speculation within the scientific community about both the root causes and the diagnosis of "leaky gut syndrome," but for the time being, research seems to indicate that gut permeability, or "leaky gut," is legitimate and associated with acne and other inflammatory or autoimmune conditions.

Leaky gut syndrome occurs when the lining of your intestine becomes damaged and allows certain chemicals and nutrients from the food you eat to "leak" into your bloodstream. These chemicals, although relatively harmless, are *not* supposed to be in the bloodstream. So, your body does what it would do for any threat – it triggers an inflammatory response.

It's easy to see why this is a problem – if an inflammatory response is being triggered every time you eat, it's nearly impossible to avoid chronic inflammation and the acne that comes with it.

But what causes leaky gut syndrome in the first place?

Usually, the intestinal lining that protects your body from these leaks becomes damaged over years due to the repeated consumption of potent antinutrients called lectins.

Most of the foods we eat have lectins in them, and in moderate doses they pose no real threat. Plants use lectins to protect themselves from being eaten in the wild – it's their best attempt to make themselves indigestible in order to fight off any predators. If a berry has potent enough lectins to make a squirrel trying to eat it sick, then the berry survives and "reproduces", so to speak.

Just about every plant or seed has lectins in it. Some of these, humans can digest extremely well, like the lectins found in most fruits and vegetables. Some of them we really can't handle, and they enter our intestine totally undigested. These undigested lectins can actually permeate, or penetrate, our intestinal wall, and enter our bloodstream. In other words, they "punch holes" in our gut, which allows chemicals to leak through into the bloodstream and trigger an acne-causing inflammatory response.

When this intestinal wall continues to become weaker and weaker, more and more foods can pass through and trigger an inflammatory response. That's why people with leaky gut syndrome may become intolerant to foods they'd otherwise be fine with – eggs, meats, certain vegetables, etc.

Thus, avoiding lectins and other antinutrients that can contribute to leaky gut syndrome is crucial for clear skin – in the diet section we'll go over all the foods to avoid if you're sensitive to lectins, or if you commonly break out after eating certain foods.

Digestive Issue #2: An Unhealthy Gut Microbiome

You've probably heard of the gut microbiome, which is the colony of microorganisms (bacteria, fungi, yeast, etc.) living in our body that aid with digestion. We *need* the gut microbiome to help break down food, absorb nutrients, and protect the body. In fact, the connection between the gut microbiome and just about every other part of our body has been explored greatly in the last several years, and it's been shown that our gut microbiome doesn't just influence how well we digest food, but also how we feel and think throughout the day.

Now, just like leaky gut, our microbiome has a huge impact on how well our body can digest certain foods – research shows that there is a very special, intimate relationship between the gut microbiome and the health of our intestines, which means that if we're not careful, an unhealthy gut microbiome can actually increase the permeability of our intestine and lead to inflammatory acne[10].

Furthermore, research also shows that a lack of diversity in the gut microbiome (oftentimes due to antibiotics) can be to blame for food intolerances that trigger inflammation-causing allergic reactions[11]. It's important to note that these allergic reactions oftentimes aren't full-blown life-or-death ordeals– they can express themselves in various ways, *including* inflammation and acne.

Lastly, an unhealthy and unbalanced gut microbiome is associated with considerably higher rates of stress, depression and anxiety, all of which can also contribute to acne[12].

It makes sense that because our gut microbiome touches just about every aspect of our health, that it is also connected to acne, but it's important to realize that research on the microbiome is an *extremely* new field of research. That's why, contrary to what you might think, I actually don't recommend taking a *ton* of probiotics or natural anti-fungal or anti-bacterial remedies to heal the gut microbiome – oftentimes this strategy can do more harm than good. We'll cover natural probiotic-rich foods in the Diet section, and later go over the select probiotics I *do* recommend in the Supplements chapter.

Digestive Issue #3: Intolerances

In addition to the two clear-cut issues above, many people have other food intolerances that might not strictly fall into one of those two categories. Maybe, for whatever reason, there are foods that you just cannot digest properly, and when you eat them your body triggers an inflammatory response. You may have a perfectly good gut microbiome and a healthy intestinal wall, but still elicit an inflammatory response – tree nut allergies in healthy individuals is a good example of this.

Because of this, I have outlined a simple protocol that we will use in the Diet section of the book to find out which foods you may be intolerant to without having to take super expensive tests.

Side Note: SIBO, Candida, and Other Fungal/Yeast/Bacterial Issues

In addition to basic gut microbiome issues, there are also more serious and severe bacterial, fungal, and yeast-related disorders that can contribute to acne. Some of these include small intestine bacterial overgrowth (SIBO), small intestinal fungal overgrowth (SIFO), and candida, amongst many others.

These are really in their own category, because they influence all three aspects of the digestive issues that can lead to acne – they can alter the gut microbiome, can increase or alter intestinal permeability, and can even lead to intolerances.

As I briefly mentioned above, treating any one of these disorders is *extremely* problematic if you don't know what you're doing – most doctors will recommend taking a round of antibiotics, which can essentially destroy colonies of beneficial bacteria, dramatically weaken the immune system[13], and of course, in the long run, lead to more acne. On the other hand, even trying to treat these issues with natural antifungals or antibacterials (oregano oil, berberine, capric acid, etc.) can also lead to challenges. While these won't do as much damage as a prescription antibiotic, these "natural" alternatives nevertheless have the potential to wipe out good bacteria and decrease overall gut health.

Many books or bloggers take a relatively haphazard approach when it comes to diagnosing and treating these extremely serious conditions. Time and time again, I've seen this process leading to forums full of individuals following certain "SIBO" protocols without even knowing if they have SIBO. They're pumping themselves full of natural antifungals and doing far more harm than good, reporting lethargy, brain fog, and difficulties digesting foods they used to be fine with, only to be met with comments about how they're going through a "detoxing" process that can't be found in any scientific literature.

That's why our approach to these ailments will be a *diet-first* approach, followed by proper testing and, if applicable, a natural anti-fungal, anti-viral, and anti-bacterial regime. But for now, don't worry about this – as I said, in any case, *diet* comes first, *even if* you wish to treat these ailments with some added medicines. We'll cover diet in great detail in the next section and have a specific Bacterial/Yeast Overgrowth Protocol you can follow in the Protocols section.

Digestive Issues Summary

In a nutshell, intolerances and digestive issues are mainly why it's so tricky to treat acne – while most people will respond relatively similarly to different insulin-spiking or inflammatory foods, many people have problems with safe foods that are low in carbs, high in nutrients, and low in inflammation-causing omega-6 fatty acids.

Time after time, I've heard from clients that cutting out a particular food was the key factor they needed to beat acne, but you'd be amazed at *which* foods it is – seemingly safe foods, like spinach, broccoli, blackberries, avocados, or even beef can cause *certain* people issues. Yes, of course, all of these people had already cut out the biggest offenders of insulin and inflammation-driven acne, including most grains, processed foods, and sugar, but still, the food that makes all the difference is often just something that you're intolerant to.

Putting It All Together: The Real Root Causes of Acne

While there are hundreds, possibly even thousands of triggers for acne, when we look at the underlying physiological mechanisms for *why* acne forms, it almost always comes through one or more of these pathways.

As an example, poor sleep is correlated with higher rates of acne[14]. Why is this? Well, sleep loss or deprivation leads to increased biomarkers of inflammation[15], insulin resistance[16], and potentially even decreased diversity of the gut microbiome[17]. Poor sleep, in itself, is a *cause* of acne only as it increases insulin resistance and inflammation, and damages our digestive system.

To really just nail the point home, let's take a look at how all three causes actually impact the biological process of acne infection and inflammation that lead to pimples:

Insulin and insulin-driven hormones cause an increase in skin cell and sebum production, which makes it more likely for pores on the skin to become clogged with oil or dead skin cells and become infected by acne bacteria. Once the bacterial infection takes place, inflammation causes the infection to become bright, red, and protruding – a pimple forms.

There are many factors that can cause inflammation, but chief among them are dietary intolerances and digestive problems, along with other inflammation-causing compounds triggered by insulin.

It's important to remember that all of the root causes act together – insulin triggers and increases biomarkers for inflammation while our gut microbiome can actually influence the amount of acne-causing insulin we release, and so on. For this reason, tackling just one of the root causes isn't going to be sufficient to get rid of acne. We need to get to the source and tackle all three issues with our diet and lifestyle.

FAQ: What about body acne?

A pretty common question that I get is, "I have acne on my shoulders/chest/back, what should I do differently?" The answer to this question is simple – "body acne", as long as it's truly acne and not dermatitis or pityrosporum folliculitis (which we'll talk about in the next paragraph), has the *exact* same root causes as facial acne.

It doesn't matter where the acne is showing up, the same biological mechanisms are still at work. The back, chest, and shoulders are particularly suspectable to acne for the same reason that the face is – there are a lot of sebum oil glands in these areas that *can* lead to acne.

Thus, the overall strategies to combat body acne that we'll go over in the subsequent sections are equally as valid for body acne. A lot of times people see body acne as something that can be taken care of topically, since the skin on the shoulders, back seems more durable and rugged, but in the past, I've found that the same general principles hold true for body acne – that overusing harsh topical products only makes body acne worse in the long run as the body overcompensates to replenish the damage done by these products.

FAQ: What about "fungal" acne? Do they have the same root causes as "regular" acne?

There has been a *lot* of talk lately about pityrosporum folliculitis, or "fungal acne", for short. The interesting thing about fungal acne is that it is technically *not* acne – acne refers to a *bacterial* infection on the surface of the skin. More specifically, an infection from a specific type of bacteria called Propionibacterium acnes, which is why we call it "acne".

Fungal "acne", on the other hand, is a *fungal* infection having to do with a naturally occurring yeast on the surface of the skin, Malassezia. There are typically two components to fungal acne: overgrowth of Malassezia on the surface of the skin, and an inflammatory response that creates the physical symptoms of fungal acne: pus-filled whiteheads and red, flakey, itchy skin.

In these regards, fungal acne is a *lot* like bacterial acne – both sebum oil and Malassezia are natural and necessary for the skin, it's only in cases where the body produces *too* much sebum or Malassezia *and* triggers an inflammatory response that they become problems.

And what causes the body to produce too much sebum or Malassezia? Generally speaking, the overuse of skincare products, a topic which we'll cover in detail in the next section. Both sebum and Malassezia are a part of the skin's own microbiome and they only become an issue when the body "overreacts" to these agents and triggers an inflammatory response.

The tactics discussed in the following sections on diet, supplements, and lifestyle, despite being originally oriented at beating bacterial acne, will also work for fungal acne because they share the same overall goal: decreasing inflammation.

Skincare products for both bacterial and fungal acne address only half of the equation – limiting sebum oil and Malassezia production on the surface of the skin. The strategies discussed in the following sections aim not only to minimize sebum and yeast production, but also to equip your body better to handle them – you can't outrun bacteria and fungi on the surface of the skin, but by changing how your immune system reacts to these compounds, you give yourself better tools to *sustainably* prevent them in the future.

Malassezia/fungal acne differs slightly from bacterial acne in a few regards, and the dietary strategies will need to be tweaked. For this reason, there is a comprehensive chapter on the subject, The Fungal Acne Protocol.

Still, I recommend *not* skipping ahead directly to this chapter, as 90% or more of the foundational tools and techniques to beat bacterial acne apply to fungal acne as well. In fact, many folks dealing with fungal acne find that the dietary tools outlined in the following chapter work just fine, not realizing until after their acne has cleared that they were originally dealing with "fungal" acne.

Chapter 3: Why Acne Products Don't Work

If you're already sold on why we need to treat acne internally, rather than externally with creams, cleansers, and masks, then you can skip this section. If you're still skeptical, this is going to be a quick overview of why the vast majority of topical solutions fail to address the *underlying* causes of acne, and why they actually make your skin worse.

The Risks of Benzoyl Peroxide

The vast majority of over-the-counter acne products on the market today use benzoyl peroxide as the primary active ingredient in their cleansers, creams, and lotions. If you walk into a drugstore and check the label of an acne product for active ingredients, the odds are good that benzoyl peroxide is at the top of the list.

Benzoyl peroxide is designed to dry out and flake off dead skin cells and kill acne bacteria before they can infect clogged pores.

It does this by using two primary mechanisms:

- Causing the skin to become dry and flake (thus removing dead skin cells)
- Killing acne bacteria on the surface of the skin

Simply put, benzoyl peroxide prevents pores from becoming blocked in the first place and kills the bacteria that is creating acne. This probably seems like this is a pretty good combination, right?

Wrong. Unfortunately, this is a short-term solution to a much deeper issue. While benzoyl peroxide does effectively eliminate acne bacteria in the short-term, the long-term risks of using benzoyl peroxide vastly outweigh the benefits.

Acne Products also Eliminate Good Bacteria and Oil on Your Skin

Remember how we talked about the "gut microbiome" in the previous chapter? Well, just like your gut, your skin has its own natural colony of good, healthy bacteria protecting it from infections, free radicals, and threats. Maintaining a healthy skin microbiome is crucial for long-term, healthy-looking skin. Furthermore, your skin also has a healthy layer of oil that protects it from outside threats, including acne.

Benzoyl peroxide is an *anti*biotic, which means it kills bacteria - while antibiotics are often good at eliminating a single strain or type of bacteria, they rarely *only* kill bad bacteria. Benzoyl peroxide can kill the good bacteria too, which makes you more suspectable to getting acne again in the future.

Furthermore, benzoyl peroxide strips the skin of its natural protective oils, which leaves your skin dry and flakey. While this is good in the short term, the minute you stop using benzoyl peroxide, you leave your skin in a considerably worse place than where you began.

The bottom line is that benzoyl peroxide is damaging to the healthy microbiome of bacteria and oil on the skin and can leave your skin less capable of healing acne on its own. Ask yourself - do you really want to be reliant on benzoyl peroxide for the rest of your life?

Acne Products Lead to More Sebum Oil, Not Less

When you use acne products with benzoyl peroxide in them, it strips the skin of sebum oil. While this might sound like a good thing, it's really quite dangerous, and can cause more acne in the long run. Sebum oil is naturally used to help moisturize and protect the skin - some sebum oil is necessary for healthy, acne-free skin.

The key is not having *too much* sebum oil and preventing sebum oil from oxidizing (going bad or rancid) by eating a healthy diet (more on that later). By drying out your skin and stripping it of sebum oil completely, your body actually overcompensates for the dryness the only way it knows - by producing even more sebum oil. This leads to a vicious cycle of needing more and more acne products to keep your skin oil at bay.

This is a key reason why acne products might work for a few weeks, and then end up creating more acne over the long run.

Acne Products Damage the Skin and Reduce the Rate of Healing

Benzoyl peroxide doesn't just strip the skin of natural oils - it strips it of essential vitamins and antioxidants it needs to fight off threats, including acne infections. One study found that applying benzoyl peroxide to the skin resulted in a 50% drop of vitamin E within the first 30 minutes[18]. Another found that it decreased levels of vitamin C on the skin by over 70%[19]. Vitamin E protects against free radicals and infections, while vitamin C helps protect against sun damage and scar healing[20].

The end result is damaged, dry, flaky skin, and acne scars that take longer to heal.

Acne Products May Generate Dangerous Free Radicals

Free radicals are highly reactive, unstable little molecules that can damage your skin's oils, proteins, and DNA[21]. Free radicals can form through a variety of ways - sometimes they're created internally, while at other times they're created by outside factors like smoking, air pollution, eating trans-fats, or in this case, putting harmful chemicals on your face.

Without an antioxidant-rich diet, free radicals are much more likely to form, and they're highly linked to acne and long-term skin damage[22]. Several studies have even found a link between benzoyl peroxide and the formation of free radicals and tumors[23]. Have you ever wondered why smokers' skin looks so aged and weak? Free radicals are partially to blame.

What does this mean for acne products? It means that not only can they cause more acne through free radicals, but they can also cause permanent, long-term damage to the skin.

Still, the case for benzoyl peroxide causing free radicals is not conclusive - we simply don't have enough evidence from our current studies to conclude that the regular use of over-the-counter grade benzoyl peroxide can cause tumors and free radicals in humans.

With that being said, the European Union has already taken steps to make benzoyl peroxide less accessible to the public by making it a prescription-grade drug.

Putting It All Together: Why You Can't Rely on Acne Products

Simply put, acne is created because of several factors:

- Too much skin oil
- Too many skin cells

- Skin cells that don't shed properly
- Skin that can't protect itself against free radicals
- Inflammation after an acne infection takes place

Most acne products work by removing your skin's natural oils and drying out the skin - but guess what? They don't address what's causing the core issues in the first place.

In addition to causing lasting damage to your skin, benzoyl peroxide won't stop your body from producing the excess sebum oil that's causing your acne in the first place. In fact, you'll likely produce even more sebum oil to overcompensate for the dryness. It also is unlikely to stop the internal mechanisms that lead to too many skin cells being produced.

On top of that, it decreases your skin's ability to protect itself against free radicals that damage and age the skin, which also slows how quickly your skin can heal.

Acne products with benzoyl peroxide are merely covering up the symptoms of acne, not treating the underlying biological mechanisms that create them.

What About Other Topical and Oral Treatments?

In general, I don't recommend relying on many topical treatments, even natural ones like aloe vera or raw honey.

I don't think that all acne products are necessarily evil (few are as damaging as benzoyl peroxide), but finding one that works for you and which works over a long period of time seems to be next to impossible, at least for me and thousands of readers on the GoodGlow blog.

What might work for a while might stop working next week. And again, we already know that the real root causes of acne lie beneath the skin. With that being said, there are a few specific types of products that I get questions about quite frequently and would like to comment on.

Salicylic acid

Salicylic acid is another popular ingredient in over-the-counter acne cleansers and creams. For starters, this is much, much better and safer than benzoyl peroxide.

Salicylic acid comes from willow tree bark, and due to its acidic properties, it unclogs pores and loosens old, dead, dry skin. This process can prevent pores from becoming blocked and acne infections taking place.

The downsides of salicylic acid are redness, irritation, and dry skin, but overall it's relatively safe. From personal experience, I've seen salicylic acid work for months, only to stop when the skin adapts to it. I'm left with damaged, red, and dry skin. While I personally believe that the skin microbiome fares better without salicylic acid, it is a much better choice than benzoyl peroxide and may be useful for minor cases of acne that don't require dietary intervention.

Oral Antibiotics

Please, please, please - don't take oral antibiotics (or topical, for that matter) to treat your acne.

Your gut flora, or the balance of bacteria in your gut, plays a huge role in making sure you digest food properly, absorb nutrients, and have a properly functioning immune system. Many dermatologists believe that by using antibiotics that aim to destroy certain strains of bacteria in the gut, you can remove the acne-causing bacteria and be left with a good-ole' happy digestive system.

This is simply incorrect.

A single dosage of oral antibiotics can permanently damage your gut microbiome. While you may experience benefits at first, the long-term damage caused by taking an oral antibiotic for acne, like tetracycline, minocycline or doxycycline, is almost certainly going to cause you more acne in the future.

I strongly believe that a large part of my own adult acne was caused by excessive antibiotic usage during my childhood and teens. Thanks, dermatologists!

Retin-A/Tretinoin

Retinoids are topical forms of vitamin A which help with the shedding of dead skin cells. They exfoliate the skin and help fight against inflammation. I think retinoids are a much safer alternative to benzoyl peroxide, but still, they're not without downsides:

- Irritation
- Swelling
- Redness
- Peeling
- Extreme sensitivity to sun exposure

Trust me, after nearly 2 years of using a low concentration of Tretinoin and still having red, inflamed, peeling skin, it's hard to say they're the cure-all. Topical retinoids may also affect your skin's ability to utilize vitamin A on its own.

Isotretinoin

Just like antibiotics, I just simply wouldn't recommend Isotretinoin as the risks vastly outweigh the benefits. Isotretinoin functions by reducing the size of the glands that produce sebum oil. It is a powerful drug that affects several major aspects of the body, not just the skin.

While this process leads to less oily, acne-prone skin, it also means your skin will be extremely dry, red, and inflamed. Without natural oils to protect the skin, extreme sensitivity to the sun and other external stimuli is common.

While Isotretinoin may be a powerful method for treating severe cases of acne, the potential side effects are equally as potent:

- Hair loss
- Heart disease
- Dry mouth
- Intracranial hypertension (increased pressure around the brain)
- Birth defects
- Depression
- Mood and energy swings

While these side effects are not extremely common, they do occur, and it's worth asking yourself if getting rid of acne is worth risking your long-term health for.

I know how badly acne can suck, but ask yourself if it's really worth losing your hair, damaging your digestive system, or altering your mood in order to get rid of it, especially when health and lifestyle changes can result in drastic transformations in skin health without the side effects.

In the Diet section, we'll actually go over how foods high in a very specific form of vitamin A can mimic many of the same acne-fighting benefits of Isotretinoin without the risks.

Sulfur & Zinc

Sulfur and zinc are two popular remedies that many online dermatology practices are now recommending.

Surprisingly, these are two topical approaches that I think are relatively harmless in the case of bacterial acne, and potentially beneficial in the case of fungal acne, granted that the sulfur and zinc products you're using have minimal added ingredients.

See The Fungal Acne Protocol for more information.

Recommended "Natural" Skincare Protocol

There will be a whole chapter on Natural Skincare in the Lifestyle & Supplements section, but I urge you to wait and read the next section, Diet, first.

There *are* useful, affordable, skin-microbiome friendly skincare alternatives to these products out there, I just firmly believe that diet, nutrition, and lifestyle should come first – otherwise you're *still* just covering up the *symptoms* of acne, albeit with gentler products.

Again, the important thing to stress here is that when you fix the internal issues that lead to acne, you won't need the expensive products you've used in the past to cover up the symptoms of the disease.

Section II: Diet

Chapter 4: Myths, Misconceptions and Mistakes

We will *never* have the scientific evidence necessary to *definitively* say that certain foods and drinks are behind all cases of acne. How certain people react to one food can be completely different than how someone else reacts. For this reason, you won't find blanket statements like, "bread causes acne" in this chapter, or any promises that cutting out a certain food will give you clear skin.

What we *do* have is a myriad of studies that demonstrate a compelling the link between how *most people* react to certain food groups and its effect on the underlying biological mechanisms that lead to acne.

In this section we'll take a look at several of these studies, homing in on particular foods and food groups, including dairy, high carbohydrate diets, chocolate, alcohol, caffeine, and dozens of others that may play a role in causing acne.

In some way, shape, or form, all of the foods that cause acne trigger one of the three root causes of acne: insulin, inflammation, or indigestion. And now that we understand the root causes of acne, it's time to dive into how you can optimize your diet to *avoid* these root causes.

Because they are all *internal*, occurring mainly in our digestive system or bloodstream, we're going to have to change our own physiology in order to beat it, and the *best* way to do that is with our diet. While supplements and lifestyle adjustments like exercise, sleep, and stress management will all play an important role, a healthy diet is *by far* the biggest step we can make towards clear skin (we'll discuss the rest later).

In the next chapter, we're going to cover the major dietary drivers of acne:

1. Foods and drinks that spike acne-causing hormones (insulin)
2. Foods and drinks that increase inflammation
3. Foods and drinks that are difficult to digest

But before we get there, we need to get rid of a few preconceived ideas you might have about starting this journey that could get in the way. These are the biggest roadblocks I've seen people encounter.

Mistake #1: Thinking That Adding "Healthier" Foods Is the Answer

Very rarely will adding a particular food or supplement to your diet help get rid of acne. The reason for this is very simple – the root causes that trigger acne can certainly be weakened by eating the right "superfoods" (e.g. anti-inflammatory foods), but in general the root causes aren't caused by nutritional deficiencies or the fact that you're not eating a certain food, they're caused by eating the wrong foods.

There are some foods you can eat that'll help blunt hormone production or inflammation, but in general, the key is to cut out foods that cause these issues in the first place.

Nutritional deficiencies, even in the age of processed foods, are relatively rare. In order to achieve success, we're going to have to stop thinking, "What superfoods should I add?" and instead think, "Which foods should I stop eating for a period of time to see if they're causing acne?"

We should look at this process not as a journey to add new foods to your diet to beat acne, but instead as a methodical approach to find out what foods that you're currently eating are causing your acne and replace them with safer foods.

That's why the entire structure of the next chapter is not around which foods you need to *add* to beat acne, but rather a complete, comprehensive breakdown of which foods trigger each of the three major causes of acne. We will go over a long list of foods at the end of this chapter, with a quick little summary on each, but this shift away from "which superfoods should I add" to "which foods do I need to test through an elimination diet" is absolutely critical.

Mistake #2: Not Understanding That Everything is Personal

Macadamia nuts are one of the safest foods out there for acne. Still, there are millions of people on the planet who have allergies to macadamia nuts that could trigger inflammatory acne. The same goes for any "safe food" or "superfood" out there.

Some people do extremely well with a diet high in saturated fat, whereas other people actually find themselves experiencing increased fungal acne while following this diet. Ruminant meat (beef, goat, etc.), on paper, at least, is a very safe food, but some people have a hard time digesting it. Cheese is generally problematic for acne, but you might find it actually helps your skin.

This is a personal journey. You need to figure out what works for you and your body. That's why in the Protocols section, we'll go over a simple, easy process to help you figure out which foods and drinks are right for *you* without expensive and inaccurate tests.

The information below is a recommendation for where to start your journey, not fixed guidelines you have to adhere to.

Mistake #3: Not Sticking With It and Setting Unrealistic Expectations

Honestly, you should start to see results pretty quickly, especially if you have rather aggressive acne – I did, and many others who read the GoodGlow blog have, at least. You'll likely notice improvements within the first few weeks. But still, while some clinical studies showed marked improvements in as little as two weeks, many others indicated that improvements generally take place over 1-3-month periods.

If your acne has formed over several years, it may take quite some time to heal, but it *will* heal, and you'll no longer have to worry about covering up the symptoms with products and pills.

It's going to be a long road, and there are going to be speedbumps and setbacks along the way. Don't get discouraged - stick with it for the long haul. If you view this change as a temporary "fix" to get rid of acne with the intention of going back to your old ways as soon as your acne's gone, it's simply not going to work. You need to truly want to make these dietary and lifestyle changes.

Similarly, don't make dietary changes that you know are going to make you miserable - at least not all at once. You're probably going to have to give up eating some of the foods you enjoy (and in the process, find new foods you enjoy, too), but that doesn't mean you have to do it all at once. Some people do better when going cold turkey, while others prefer weaning themselves off. Be kind to yourself and do whatever you have to do to make lasting changes.

Find foods that don't make you break out which you enjoy. There are probably dozens of foods you've never tried before that are great for your skin and taste great.

How to read this section

The structure of this section is going to be pretty straightforward: we'll go over which types of food and food groups trigger the three root causes of acne. This will be our broad overview of the diet, so that you can understand *why* you should avoid certain foods. Then, we'll do a quick summary of over 100 foods and drinks so that that you can quickly and easily identify which foods will work for you. Finally, we'll move onto some practical advice on how to avoid acne-causing foods while shopping, eating out, etc.

Chapter 5: Foods That Trigger Acne's Root Causes

Now is when we get to the fun stuff – it's time to start tying together what we've learned in the Root Causes section and apply it to our diet. We know what the underlying biological mechanisms of acne are – hormones, inflammation, and digestive issues. Now we can ask, "What foods and drinks cause these issues?"

We'll break it down one by one, and bear in mind that there's going to be some *big* overlap here. We'll go over each food group (and summaries for over 100 foods/drinks) in the next chapter, but this will act as a guiding principle for *why* you should avoid certain foods or drinks.

Remember – our key focus for clear skin is *not* adding super foods or supplements, but rather *avoiding* the key drivers of acne.

1. Foods and Drinks that Spike Acne-Causing Hormones (Insulin)

We've already covered the basics of insulin, so I'll be brief in summarizing it here: insulin is a hormone that the body releases to help convert sugar in the bloodstream into usable energy for the body. Insulin isn't evil, but when *too much* insulin is triggered, it leads to the overproduction of skin cells and sebum oil, inflammation, and eventually acne.

But what foods trigger the most insulin?

In general, it's safe to summarize that *carbohydrate-rich* foods trigger the largest insulin spikes. The reason for this is pretty straightforward – all the carbohydrates you eat *eventually* turn into sugar in the bloodstream and need to be converted into glycogen (usable energy).

Protein-heavy foods also increase insulin levels, but typically to a lesser degree, while fat-heavy foods have little-to-no effect on insulin levels (as fat can be used directly for energy) and sometimes even blunt the insulin-producing effect of other foods.

In general, more carbohydrates mean more insulin, which means a higher likelihood of hormonal acne.

So, does that mean you should just totally avoid carbs? Absolutely not. *Where* you get your carbs from makes a *huge* difference in the amount of insulin that your body produces.

You might have heard of "simple" versus "complex" carbs, or "fast" versus "slow" carbs, and these distinctions make a pretty large difference in how our bodies metabolize food and trigger insulin responses. Different foods, despite having similar numbers of carbs, generally elicit very different, very unique insulin responses. The reason for this is that there are three main types of carbohydrates, each of which trigger a different insulin response from the body:

- Sugars – carbs that are quickly converted into energy the body can use
- Starches – carbs that take longer to be converted into energy the body can use
- Fiber – carbs that your body can't digest and therefore can't use for energy

With the exception of fiber, your body breaks down *all* carbohydrates into glucose. Glucose is used by your brain and your muscles to carry out their necessary functions. The ratio of these three types of carbohydrates, along with how much fat and protein a food has, all influence the severity of the insulin spike that comes from the food.

Foods high in sugar and low in fiber and starches typically trigger rapid, large insulin responses from the body. Conversely, foods with a lot of fiber or starch will typically have a lower insulin response from the body, making them far safer for our skin.

Scientists have tested various foods and their general insulin responses and come up with different measurements or benchmarks to explain this. Maybe you've heard of the glycemic index (GI), glycemic load (GL), or insulin index. These are all ways of explaining what type of effect this food will have on blood sugar and/or insulin levels.

We'll be using these measurements to get an idea of which carbohydrate sources and foods are most likely to trigger acne.

High-GI List: Insulin-Spiking Foods

Below is a table that contains the glycemic index of various foods. Basically, the higher the GI, the more rapidly a food spikes your blood sugar (and consequently, the more likely it is to trigger acne-causing insulin). While it's impossible to get this data on *every* food, this chart will act as an initial starting place for us. Foods with a glycemic index of greater than 70 are considered dangerous, high-GI foods. Foods between 55 and 70 are in the middle zone, and foods below 55 are considered low-GI.

Food	Glycemic Index

Food	Glycemic Index
GRAINS AND STARCHES	
Wheat bread	75
Corn tortilla	46
White rice	73
Brown rice	68
Sweet corn	52
Spaghetti	49
Instant oatmeal	79
Biscuits	69
Cornflakes	81
Baked russet potato	111
Boiled white potato	82
Instant mashed potato	87
Sweet potato	70
Yam	54
Sweet corn	60
Quinoa	53
White rice	89
Brown rice	50
Cereal	77
Cornflakes	93
Instant oatmeal	83
Graham crackers	74
Vanilla wafers	77
Shortbread	64
DAIRY	
Ice cream, regular	57
Milk, full fat	41
Reduced-fat yogurt with fruit	33
FRUITS	

Food	Glycemic Index
Apple	39
Banana, ripe	62
Dates, dried	42
Grapefruit	25
Grapes	59
Orange	40
Peach	42
Pear	38
Prunes, pitted	29
Raisins	64
Watermelon	72
BEANS AND NUTS	
Baked beans	40
Blackeye peas	33
Black beans	30
Chickpeas	10
Navy beans	31
Kidney beans	29
Lentils	29
Soy beans	15
Cashews	27
Peanuts	7
SNACK FOODS	
Corn chips, plain, salted	42
Fruit Candy	99
Microwave popcorn, plain	55
Potato chips	51
Pretzels, oven-baked	83
Chocolate Bar	51
VEGETABLES	

Food	Glycemic Index
Green peas	51
Carrots	35
Parsnips	52
BEVERAGES	
Soda	59
Apple juice	41
Cranberry juice	68
Sports drink	78
Orange juice	50
Tomato juice	38

Source: Harvard Health, The University of Sydney

It's worth noting that this table is *not* the only measure for whether a food will cause insulin-driven acne (dairy has a low GI but triggers a *ton* of insulin, which we'll talk about in a bit*)*, but it acts as a good guide to get started from when understanding which foods are likely causing hormonal acne.

What can we learn from this table?

Well, there are a few takeaways…

Avoid High-Sugar Foods (Most Fruit is Fine, Though)

Have you ever found yourself breaking out after binging on some sweets? The reason for this is pretty simple – sugar, or rather two particular types of sugar, glucose and sucrose, are *extremely* insulinogenic.

Upon entering the body, both forms of simple sugar can enter the bloodstream without a hefty conversion process (glucose is what is used in the body anyway), so the insulin spike is rapid and immediate, *especially* in the absence of fiber or fats that can help blunt the insulin spike.

That's why sweets, desserts, and high-sugar foods are some of the worst foods you can possibly eat for acne. This includes things like sports drinks (which claim to contain electrolytes) which are really just overpriced sugar water. In reality, just about *anything* with more than a few grams of *added* sugar, which is almost always glucose, sucrose, or an analogous, insulin-spiking alternative, should be avoided for this very simple reason.

In nature, foods with this amount of added sugar and little to no fiber simply don't exist. Fruits that are naturally high in sugar, like apples, also contain fiber to blunt the insulin spike, for instance. Luckily, it's now required on nutrition labels to disclose the amount of "added" sugar in food products, so be aware that your favorite nutrition bar or energy booster might actually be an acne-causing machine.

There is one important caveat here – *fructose*, a form of sugar commonly found in fruit, has about one-third the glycemic index of sucrose and glucose, making it considerably safer for your skin in moderate amounts.

Plus, as previously mentioned, many fruits contain fiber to offset the insulin spike of the naturally occurring sugar found in fruit. As you can see in the chart above, and as we'll go over in further detail in the next section, there are some fruits that are better than others in this regard, but for the most part, fruits are exceptions to the "sugar is bad" rule. That does *not* include fruit juices, which contain no fiber and which are therefore basically glorified sugar water.

Most Starches

One thing that might surprise you is that some starches, like yams, have a ton of carbs but a *relatively* modest glycemic index. Why, for example, is the glycemic index of a yam so much less than the glycemic index of a potato? Why is brown rice lower than white rice?

In general, starches have a lower glycemic index than sugar, because starches contain both fiber and complex carbohydrates that need to be broken down into glucose, thus delaying the insulin spike.

Starches with more fiber, like yams and brown rice, have more mechanisms in place to slow down the insulin spike versus something like potatoes (without the skin) or white rice.

With that being said, it's extremely important to note (as we'll cover in the next section) that this difference is relatively negligible, at least in the case of something like white rice versus brown rice, and that optimizing your diet for easier digestion is almost always more important than optimizing for a lower insulin spike when it comes to acne.

For now, the takeaway is simple: most starches spike insulin considerably, and while not all carbs are evil, we need to put starches on our radar when we go about forming a plan to beat acne. Depending on our body's insulin sensitivity, we might need to cut back on the starches for a period of time.

Dairy

If you paid close attention to the glycemic index chart, you're probably wondering why I recommend cutting out (most) dairy. It's low in carbs and has a low glycemic index, so it shouldn't trigger a big insulin spike, right? Wrong.

Because dairy, unlike many other foods, contains particular proteins (casein, whey) in addition to carbohydrates (lactose) that spike insulin, it appears to be insulin-safe but really is quite problematic. Beef protein, for instance, isn't very insulinogenic. But casein and whey, two of the primary proteins found in dairy, along with lactose, the primary carbohydrate found in dairy, create the ultimate trigger for insulin production.

Insulin: The Takeaway

When it comes to hormonal acne, nothing is more important than insulin and its acne-causing friends, IG-1, IGFBP-3, and IL-1. The foods that spike insulin generally fall into three camps: high-sugar foods (excluding fruit), starches, and dairy.

Again, in the next section you'll get the whole rundown on exactly what foods to keep in mind when it comes to insulin.

Foods and drinks that increase inflammation

Inflammation is a tricky subject, because so many different factors influence it. For this particular section, I'd like to hone in on one major source of dietary-driven inflammation that's rampant, and that's the overconsumption of omega-6 fatty acids.

Again, we've already covered this, so I'll give the quick summary here: omega fatty acids have a powerful effect on our immune system and our body's inflammatory response. Omega-3 fatty acids, like those found in fish, have an anti-inflammatory effect, meaning that they help prevent the biological mechanisms that cause acne. Omega-6 fatty acids, on the other hand, which are found in *tons* of food, have an inflammatory effect, meaning they lend themselves more to acne.

Omega-6 fatty acids are found all over the place, and until

recently they weren't a huge problem – we used to eat approximately an equal amount of omega-3 and omega-6, but as consumption of wild-caught seafood decreased and consumption of seed and vegetable oils increased, this started to tip rapidly in the other direction, to the point where it's now roughly 20 to 1 in favor of omega-6.

So, what foods and drinks are driving this massive increase, and causing inflammation-driven acne?

Vegetable and Seed Oils

The main dietary driver for this is vegetable and seed oils. These oils, which include soybean oil, wheat germ oil, corn oil, sesame oil, peanut oil, cottonseed oil, grapeseed oil, flaxseed oil, sunflower oil, margarine, shortening, and canola oil, are all *loaded* with omega-6 fatty acids. Traditionally, these oils were difficult to extract, but with modern food processing technology we can extract oil from soybeans with little difficulty, even though nature never quite intended it. Compare that process to something like olive oil (which contains a fraction of the omega-6 content) and bear in mind that producing olive oil has been done for thousands of years, and you can get a basic idea for how foreign this concept of squeezing seeds for oil really is.

Here's a list of healthy, low omega-6 fats and oils and their omega-6 content:

Food	Omega-6 Per Serving (mg)
Olive Oil	1400
Avocado oil	1754
Ghee	300

Butter	382
Coconut Oil	243
Tallow	168

Now, here's a short list of vegetable oils and their omega-6 content:

Food	Omega-6 Per Serving (mg)
Canola Oil	
Corn Oil	5270
Grape Seed Oil	14944
Margarine	9744
Safflower Oil	6128
Soy Oil	10447
Sunflower Oil	14192
Shortening	9198

Notice how these vegetable oils contain 5-10x the amount of omega-6 as our healthy oils? It's really something to think about - a single tablespoon of one of these dangerous oils contains more omega-6 than our ancestors would have likely consumed over the course of a single day. Now, you might be thinking to yourself, "Great, but I only use olive oil at home," or something like that, and I'd like to caution you because the *majority* of processed, packaged foods contain these vegetable oils.

Protein, nutrition and "health" bars, salad dressings, dips, cookies, sauces, trail mix, chips, many roasted nuts, and a whole assortment of other foods contain these oils in pretty large doses, and as we've seen, it doesn't take much of them to cause inflammation. Additionally, many restaurants, particularly fast food restaurants, will use vegetable oils in favor of healthy fats.

For this reason, reading nutrition labels and avoiding these oils is crucial.

Fried Foods

Fried foods, like French fries, calamari, chicken tenders, etc., are all loaded with omega-6 fatty acids because they're fried in vegetable oils. Worse yet, the vegetable oils are oxidated at these extremely high temperatures, making them even more damaging to your overall health.

Fried foods are one of the few categorically bad groups of food when it comes to your health and your skin.

Nuts and Seeds (in Large Amounts)

Many, and in fact most, nuts and seeds are high in omega-6 fatty acids. Refer to the following list to get a better idea:

Food	Omega-6 Per Ounce (mg)
Almonds	3378
Cashews	2178
Chia Seeds	1619
Coconut	102
Flax Seeds	1655
Hazelnuts	2192
Hemp Seeds	7660
Pecans	5776

Food	Omega-6 Per Ounce (mg)
Pistachios	3696
Pumpkin Seeds	2452
Sunflower Seeds	5984
Walnuts	10666
Macadamia Nuts	370

This does *not* mean that you need to avoid these foods, as in fact many of them are loaded with acne-fighting nutrients and are also great low-carb fuel sources that won't spike insulin, but rather that you should use them in moderation, as a snack (I know, it's hard not to have too much!) Some of them, like walnuts, you may want to avoid due to the simply *massive* amount of omega-6.

It's also worth noting that while peanuts are technically a legume, they contain an *insane* amount of omega-6, and should just generally be avoided.

Others

There are a lot of seemingly random foods which are high in omega-6 that you probably wouldn't expect. Again, there will be a breakdown of hundreds of foods in the following section, but here's a short primer:

- Chicken skin, thighs, wings
- Bacon
- Tofu
- Many soups
- Some eggs (varies greatly depending on diet/variety – commercial eggs are much higher in omega-6)

Summary: Inflammation

The name of the game when it comes to inflammation-driven acne is avoiding vegetable and seed oils. Yes, there are other foods that are relatively high in omega-6, but if you can cut these out, you're 90% of the way there.

Foods and drinks that are difficult to digest

This is going to sound like quite the controversial statement (and I'll back it up in a second), but foods that are difficult to digest are *almost always* plant-based food. Why? Because digestive difficulties typically stem from eating antinutrients, which are compounds that plants (and *only* plants) produce in order to survive.

Things, whether they're plants or animals, do not like to be eaten. Every organism on the planet has natural defensive mechanisms in order to defend itself from predators and pass its genes onto the next generation. Animals can run, flee, fight, and hide. These are their primary mechanisms of defense. Plants, on the other hand, (typically) cannot use movement or evasive action to survive. Instead, they need to develop their own defensive mechanisms which will prevent animals, whether a squirrel or a human, from eating them. These are called antinutrients, and they're the root of most digestive issues that trigger autoimmune conditions and food intolerances that lead to acne.

Now, before we even start to talk about which plant-based foods this occurs most in, I feel extremely obligated to say that *plants are not evil*, and in fact the current scientific consensus is that most antinutrients, eaten *in moderation,* are beneficial. Much like how exercise-induced physical stress increases the performance and health of the body overall, a little bit of stress from these antinutrients may be beneficial.

With that being said, there are a few *key* antinutrients that are either flat-out damaging, even in small amounts, or antinutrients that in *larger* doses can be quite problematic, especially for acne.

Typically, a person will have a hard time tolerating a certain set of antinutrients, rather than *all* plant-based antinutrients.

Our strategy is to figure out what these antinutrients are, which foods contain them, and whether or not we can *personally* tolerate these antinutrients. Some people may have no issue with high levels of phytic acid, for instance, while struggling immensely with oxalates. We will cover how to figure this out in a following section, but for now let's break down the biggest and most dangerous antinutrients and which foods contain them.

Lectins & Gluten

Lectins are antinutrients that plants use to prevent predators from eating them – they're designed to harm the digestive system of the animals (and humans) who eat them. We've evolved to be able to eat and tolerate a wide range of lectins, and in many cases, small doses of lectins don't really do a lot of damage.

During the digestive process, lectins are not broken down like they should be. They stay intact and float down to the intestine, where they actually pass through the intestinal lining fully intact. Once they're in your bloodstream, your body sees them as a threat and sends out an inflammatory response as if the lectin were a harmful bacterium or a virus – in essence, if your body is sensitive to lectins, they will trigger an inflammatory response, and likely, inflammatory acne.

Grains, like wheat, are extremely high in lectins. Aside from your typical lectin, gluten is a particularly damaging plant protein. It's a huge part of the reason why so many people have a hard time digesting grain. Some research suggests that even if you don't have a gluten intolerance, the lectins found in bread can still trigger acne-causing inflammation[24]. Still, all other grains contain lectins too, of varying amounts and severities.

Beans and legumes are also huge sources of lectins, which, in addition to their high phytic acid content, makes them extremely problematic for many individuals struggling with acne.

Lectins are actually the reason why white rice, despite its high glycemic index, is a better choice for acne than brown rice – the lectins within rice are found in the hull, which is removed in the process of making white rice. While I don't necessarily recommend you pick up white rice as a dietary staple, it's a very easy food to digest for this reason.

Dairy and eggs also contain lectins, in varying amounts, making them stand out against meat and seafood which don't contain lectins.

The key with lectins is to avoid *high-lectin* foods – unless you adopt the Carnivore Protocol, you simply won't be able to avoid *all* lectins. Here are the biggest contributors to watch out for:

- Grains (barley, buckwheat, millet, quinoa, rye, wheat, oats, brown/wild rice) and any products made with grain or grain flour
- Legumes (lentils, chickpeas, beans, etc.)
- White potatoes
- Peanuts and peanut-based products
- Some dairy in high amounts (milk, kefir, sour cream, ice cream, cheese)
- Corn and corn-based products
- Tomatoes
- Beer
- Some nuts and seeds in *large* amounts (cashews)

Phytic Acid/Phytate

Phytic acid is an antinutrient found in grains, legumes, nuts, and other plant-based foods that prevents you from properly absorbing nutrients like iron, zinc, calcium, manganese, copper, and magnesium. This is particularly problematic for acne – manganese, magnesium, and *especially zinc*, are all critical for clear skin.

Phytic acid is a huge factor when it comes to how much zinc you actually your body actually absorbs[25]. Many beans and legumes are extremely high in phytic acid, which isn't problematic if you're eating them in moderation (phytic acid can actually fight acne-causing free radicals in small doses), but in higher amounts could lead to nutritional deficiencies.

As a whole, excess phytic acid is something we want to avoid because it prevents us from being able to absorb the nutrients our body needs to actually fight acne.

The good news is that by properly cooking your food, you can minimize the amount of phytic acid in *most* foods by a considerable amount.

Here are the largest contributors to watch out for:

- All grains
- All legumes (lentils, garbanzo beans, etc.)
- Raw dark, leafy vegetables (especially spinach, chard, and kale)
- Dark chocolate
- Nuts and seeds in high amounts
- Peanuts

Oxalates

Oxalates are antinutrients that bind to calcium in the blood and which can lead to things like kidney stones or inflammation. While kidney stones are not good, we'll focus on the inflammation aspect of oxalates because this directly pertains to acne.

Oxalates are a highly debated and contentious topic in the world of antinutrients. Some nutritionists and experts claim that oxalates present little to no health risks, while others (especially in the carnivore diet community) claim that they're among the *most* damaging. One study found that oxalates may be responsible for, "A wide variety of other health problems related to inflammation, auto-immunity, mitochondrial dysfunction, mineral balance, connective tissue integrity, urinary tract issues and poor gut function"[26].

I can personally say that adopting a low-oxalate diet has made a difference for me and my skin, as well as for many of my readers, but one of the largest issues with oxalates is the sheer number of foods that contain them.

Kale, spinach, and chard, all seemingly healthy "superfoods," all contain extremely high amounts of oxalate. Beans, beer, berries, chocolate, coffee, tea, and other dark green vegetables are all major sources, too.

In fact, when you *really* look into the issue, it almost seems as if only some fruit, meat, and seafood are on the table when it comes to low-oxalate foods. I don't think this is a sustainable or necessary approach for most people, so I think that focusing on cutting down on the highest oxalate foods is the best strategy.

- Avoid *raw* dark leafy vegetables (especially kale, chard, and spinach – always lightly cook these vegetables to minimize oxalates)
- All legumes/beans

- Beer
- Chocolate
- Coffee
- Black tea

Summary: Anti-nutrients

There are hundreds of other antinutrients we didn't even begin to cover here, but the three that I'd like to stress are lectins (and gluten), phytic acid, and oxalates. These seem to be, from both clinical literature and personal experience helping others, the three largest antinutrients behind acne.

It's important to realize that it's not necessary to completely cut out these antinutrients (unless you *really* want to – see the Carnivore Protocol) but rather to minimize them by cutting out the largest offenders. This includes:

- All grains (with the exception of white rice in some cases)
- All corn
- All legumes/beans (including peanuts)
- *Raw* dark leafy vegetables (especially kale, chard, and spinach – always lightly cook these vegetables to minimize anti-nutrients)
- Beer

You'll likely want to limit or closely watch your consumption of the following foods when it comes to anti-nutrients:

- Nuts and seeds
- Coffee
- Tea
- Dark chocolate

We'll cover specifically which foods you might want to avoid due to antinutrients in the next chapter.

Summary: The 3 Dietary Drivers of Acne

Now we've got a pretty good overview of the primary dietary drivers of acne. In a nutshell, we can summarize them as follows:

- Insulin: high-sugar foods, most starches, and most dairy
- Inflammation: vegetable and seed oils, fried foods, some nuts and seeds
- Digestion: grains, legumes, corn, and *potentially* some vegetables, nuts, coffee, and tea

Now just looking at that list, you might start thinking to yourself, "What *is* safe to eat, just meat, seafood, and fruit?" This *is not* a list of foods that you need to avoid – this is just a broad outline that can act as a starting place for where to begin your own clear skin diet.

The overwhelming majority of people do *not* have to substantially limit their diet. In fact, more often than not, eliminating one of the three drivers is all that's needed for clear skin, but it's still important to understand the holistic relationship between diet and acne before jumping into particular foods.

Speaking of which, now we can finally jump into the fun stuff – a comprehensive food list.

Chapter 6: Clear Skin Food List

In this section, we'll break down which foods are most likely to give you issues when it comes to acne. In the spirit of the previous section, we'll be avoiding labeling anything a "superfood" (with the notable exception of wild-caught seafood and organ meats, which we'll cover soon) and instead focus on the foods that are *most likely* to be causing dietary-driven acne.

For each of the individual foods, we'll also have a short rating next to it:

- **Safe**: this food is *generally* safe for your skin
- **Unsafe**: this food is *generally* problematic for acne, and you should probably cut it out if you can
- **Limit**: this food probably isn't likely to cause acne in small amounts, but you want to be careful
- **Test it**: this food is probably fine, but it contains some compounds that may cause acne in certain individuals, so you do want to test it
- **It depends:** certain types of this food might be safe for your skin, while others might not. For example, white rice is generally safe, while brown rice is not.

You can use this rating to get a quick idea of which foods to avoid and which ones are safe, but I still highly recommend reading through the entire section so that you have an idea of *why* you might want to avoid certain foods.

Once you have all the knowledge you need, we'll go over the practicalities of making this a reality by planning out your own personal diet.

A Note About "Unsafe" Foods

Notice how I'm purposely labeling foods that are likely to cause acne as "unsafe" rather than "foods to avoid"? There's a reason for this - this list *isn't* a definitive answer of what foods you need to cut out of your diet.

Depending on genetic, hormonal, and lifestyle factors, you might be able to indulge in some, or many, of these foods without any problems. Rather, you should look at these foods as a starting place for refining your diet – if you want to start making changes in the direction of eating a clean diet for clear skin, these are the most obvious foods and food groups to start with.

I'll point out the healthier options in each food group – for instance, when it comes to starches and grains, sweet potatoes are usually a pretty good choice over bread, but I'm not here to tell you that you *have* to cut out bread. These are all simply starting places for foods you should consider cutting out.

Without further ado, let's jump right in...

Grains & Starches

Most grains (breads, cereals, corn, pasta, etc.) are a nightmare for acne for two reasons: they are almost all high in carbohydrates, which triggers a large insulin response from the body and can lead to insulin-driven hormonal acne, and they contain high amounts of antinutrients which can damage the digestive system and lead to inflammatory acne. Furthermore, many people have specific food sensitivities to the compounds found in many grains, triggering an inflammatory response that can lead to acne.

Unsafe: Wheat

For the vast majority of people, wheat is the most problematic grain because it contains extremely damaging antinutrients (gluten) as well as short-chain fermentable carbohydrates that trigger a large insulin and inflammation response. The type of wheat doesn't really make a considerable difference here – white, wheat, sourdough, etc. - are all potential issues if you struggle with acne-prone skin. I generally recommend cutting out wheat during the elimination period and adding it back in later if you must.

Unsafe: Corn

Corn isn't as damaging as wheat, but if you've ever looked at your stool after eating corn, you can tell that it's a challenge for the body to digest. It contains a lectin called zein which can trigger inflammatory acne, and it's very high in carbohydrates which can lead to inflammatory acne.

Unsafe: Rye/Buckwheat

Rye also contains gluten and has a high glycemic index. Buckwheat does not contain gluten but has other lectins which can act like gluten in the body. For most people I've worked with, buckwheat and rye aren't as damaging as wheat and intolerances aren't quite as common, but I still wouldn't recommend adding it if you can avoid it.

Test it: Quinoa

Compared to other grains, quinoa is a generally safe grain. It contains a lectin called prolamine, which can cause issues similar to gluten in sensitive individuals, but which is nowhere near as problematic. It's still pretty high in carbs, but I'd say it's one of the safer options here. If you don't have a reason to eat it, I'd recommend avoiding it just to be safe, but if you enjoy quinoa and cut it out for several weeks and notice no changes, consider adding it back.

Limit: Oats

Again, oats don't have gluten, but they have something that's close – avenin. This can cause digestive-driven inflammation which can contribute to acne. They're also high in carbs and phytic acid, which means your body won't be able to properly absorb the acne-fighting nutrients you need for clear skin (like zinc). As a whole, I'd recommend avoiding or cutting out if you can.

It depends: Rice

Not all rice is created equal. While a lot of people tend to see brown rice as a healthier alternative to white rice, the truth of the matter is that brown, wild, and other non-white types of rice all contain a significant amount of antinutrients. This is because the husk, the outside shell of the rice, is where most of the antinutrients are found. By stripping off the husk (and thus making white rice), you eliminate most of the antinutrients, but at a small cost – less fiber, which means a greater insulin spike.

White rice is a pretty safe, easily digestible choice for acne, but because of its high glycemic index, I'd recommend using with caution if you struggle with insulin-driven acne. Still, its easily digestible nature makes it a better choice than brown or wild rice for most people.

Safe Starches: Sweet potatoes, squash, pumpkin, yam, cassava

"Safe starches" are starches (typically root vegetables) that differ from other grains or roots because of their low antinutrient count. While most starches are high in lectins, phytic acid, or other antinutrients, these starches are *very low in antinutrients* besides oxalates, which is generally only a problem in large doses:

- Sweet potatoes (also extremely high in retinol vitamin A, which can help fight acne)
- Squash
- Pumpkin
- Yam
- Cassava

What "safe" does *not* mean is that you should be eating them all the time – all of these foods are *still* high in carbs and can still cause insulin-driven acne if you're not careful.

Safe: Sweet potatoes

Yes, I know I just had sweet potatoes in the "Safe Starches" area above, but I feel like it's extra important to bring attention to this amazing carb source. While sweet potatoes are relatively high in carbs and glycemic index, they're also loaded with an extremely high amount of vitamin A, even in beta carotene form. Vitamin A is crucial for just about every stage of the skin-clearing process, from decreasing insulin resistance to preventing inflammation, and even wound healing of acne scars *after* your skin clears. Test them out, for sure, but sweet potatoes are usually a great choice.

Limit: White potatoes

White potatoes are a high glycemic index food, which means they'll likely cause insulin-driven acne in sensitive individuals. Furthermore, they're a nightshade, which means they can cause inflammation in individuals who are sensitive. Lastly, they're relatively high in lectins, which can damage the gut. Still, they're probably not as damaging as wheat or many other grains. They don't have many nutrients so I wouldn't recommend *adding* them to your diet if you don't already eat them, but don't stress over them too much either.

Beans & legumes

Beans and legumes are a lot like grains in the sense that they are likely to cause inflammation and gut issues due to high concentrations of antinutrients, including lectins, phytic acid, and saponin (a soap-like antinutrient that can punch holes in the gut and increase intestinal permeability). Plus, like many grains, legumes also contain FODMAPs - carbohydrates that can be difficult to digest.

On the plus side, most beans and legumes have a very low glycemic index, which means they are unlikely to trigger insulin-driven hormonal acne. Despite being high in carbohydrates they also have tons of fiber, which slows down the body's insulin response.

Furthermore, proper preparation of beans and legumes can decrease their antinutrient content. Legumes have been consumed for thousands of years, and our ancestors went through great efforts to ensure that the legumes they were eating were properly prepared – research shows that we should do the same. Simply cooking legumes for as little as 15 minutes can wipe out most of the lectins they contain[27], and by soaking legumes at room temp for 18 hours you can eliminate upwards of 70% of their phytic acid content[28].

While legumes are never an amazing choice, properly prepared legumes are a *lot* safer.

Test it: Chickpeas (garbanzo beans) and Lentils (soaked

and cooked properly)

Chickpeas and lentils, if soaked and cooked properly, are two of the safest legume choices for acne-prone skin, but still not amazing selections.

Both chickpeas and lentils are effective at reducing blood sugar, and are high in fiber, manganese, and several other nutrients. Furthermore, they have about half the amount of antinutrients, including phytic acid and saponins, when compared to many other legumes, like soy and navy beans.

They also contain a large amount of zinc, which may help offset the zinc lost due to the phytic acid content of legumes. For this reason, chickpeas and lentils should *not* be used to make up for a zinc deficiency but are still safer options than other beans and legumes that are lower in zinc.

Limit: Black beans, pinto beans, kidney beans, navy beans (soaked and cooked properly)

All of these beans are moderately high in antinutrients, and from what I've experienced while running one of the leading diet-focused acne resources for the last several years, more likely to give people digestive or intolerance issues.

Generally, they have less beneficial nutrients when compared to lentils or chickpeas, so they're not worth the risk.

Properly prepared, I don't think that any of them are the worst things you could eat for acne; however, I think that you most certainly have safer carbohydrate options, which we will cover shortly.

Unsafe: Soy, soy sauce, soybeans

Soy is particularly problematic for acne-prone skin for a few reasons. First, while all beans and legumes have phytic acid, the phytic acid found in soy isn't easily destroyed even after sprouting, soaking, and cooking[29]. This prevents your body from absorbing zinc, a crucial acne-fighting nutrient.

Furthermore, there is ongoing speculation amongst researchers about whether soy causes hormonal imbalances that can lead to acne. It's believed that soy's phytoestrogens bind to estrogen receptors and mimic your body's naturally occurring estrogen without producing any of the benefits – if you're struggling specifically with hormonal acne, it might be a good idea to cut out soy.

Unsafe: Peanuts (see nuts)

Peanuts are technically a legume, but I've included them in the "Nuts & Seeds" food group section, as most people consider peanuts to be a nut. Please see that entry for more information on why peanuts are not safe for acne-prone individuals.

Dairy

With the exception of ghee, butter, and possibly a few other choice foods, most dairy is problematic for acne sufferers due to the large number of acne-causing hormones and various inflammation-causing compounds found in dairy.

Dairy is a byproduct of milk, and whether the milk is from a cow, sheep or goat, its biological purpose is to help newborns grow. To do this, milk contains hormones that trigger growth. That's good news if you're a newborn calf (or human), but not so good if you're a young adult struggling with acne. The specific hormones that dairy triggers are the very same compounds responsible for causing acne: IGF-1 and IGFBP-3.

In the previous section we went over in detail about how each of these compounds contributes to acne, but just as a quick reminder, we know that IGF-1 triggers the skin to overproduce skin cells, which rise to the surface and clog pores, that IGFBP-3 prevents the skin from shedding dead skin cells properly.

Not only does dairy *contain* a bunch of acne-causing hormones, but it also triggers your body to produce a ton of acne-causing hormones, including insulin. While dairy is safe on paper (it's low in carbs, and carbs are what triggers insulin, right?), most dairy (besides butter and some creams/cheeses) are an exception to the rule – dairy, despite being low in carbs, triggers a huge, acne-causing insulin release.

Dairy is also extremely difficult to digest. Most people are unable to properly digest a certain protein found in many dairy products - casein A1. Studies show that casein A1 can lead to inflammation, slow digestion, and aggravate symptoms of lactose intolerance.

Lastly, dairy is the single most common food intolerance on the planet, with intolerance to both dairy carbohydrates (lactose) and protein (casein A1) being extremely common. It's estimated that nearly 70% of the world's population has an issue absorbing lactose.[30]

There are plenty of reasons to avoid dairy, but that doesn't necessarily mean that you have to. In fact, there are a few sources of dairy that are actually *great* for clear skin, assuming you can tolerate them. Testing is key with dairy – try eliminating all dairy for 3-4 weeks, and then adding in certain dairy, starting with the safest options.

Safe: Ghee butter

Ghee is *by far* the safest form of dairy for acne. Ghee is simply pure butterfat, which means it doesn't have any whey, casein, or lactose. This means that it sidesteps all the major issues of dairy: ghee won't trigger any significant insulin response, contains very few omega-6 fatty acids, has plenty of antioxidants, and is stable at high temperatures. Ghee stands alongside coconut oil, extra-virgin olive oil, beef tallow, and avocado oil when it comes to safe, healthy, and effective fats.

Safe: Butter

Butter, especially if it's grass-fed, is almost as good as grass-fed ghee, except it contains small amounts of casein and lactose. Overall, these small amounts shouldn't be enough to cause massive issues, but if you're sensitive to dairy then they can still pose some challenges for acne-prone skin.

Test it: Heavy cream (full-fat, preferably raw)

Heavy cream is low in lactose, low in protein (casein and whey), and even low in omega-6 fatty acids that contribute to inflammation. The only big negative with heavy cream is that it'll still have IGF-1 in it; otherwise it's a relatively healthy fat. Again, it's not as good as ghee (or butter) in this regard, but it isn't necessarily bad.

Test it: Kefir

Kefir is a fermented dairy beverage that has a lot of commonalities with yogurt. Kefir is better for your skin than yogurt for a few reasons:

- It has more strains of probiotics than yogurt
- It's lower in lactose, omega-6 fatty acids, and protein than yogurt

- It's high in retinol (vitamin A)

Unfortunately, kefir isn't perfect – it still has some IGF-1, casein, whey, and calcium. For this reason, kefir ranks higher than other dairy products but still isn't as safe as other alternatives like ghee or butter.

Unsafe: Milk

Milk's extremely high in lactose, casein, calcium, and whey, and is extremely insulinogenic, which means it pretty much checks every box when it comes to causing acne.

There's nothing found in milk that you can't get from other foods, which is why it's generally best to just stay away from milk. If you *need* to drink some kind of milk, I'd recommend coconut or almond milk as an alternative.

If you insist on drinking milk, go for raw, organic, grass-fed milk whenever you can, and make sure you avoid skimmed milk.

Unsafe: Cheese

Pretty much all cheese contains significant amounts of casein and whey, proteins that trigger inflammation and damage the digestive system, making it generally unsafe for acne-prone skin. However, many kinds of cheese are considerably lower in lactose and IGF-1 than other cheeses. In general, aged cheeses contain less IGF-1 and more nutrients (like vitamin A) than young cheeses. Here's a list of attributes to consider when it comes to cheese:

- Goat and sheep cheeses are generally better than cow
- Aged cheese has less IGF-1 than young cheese
- Cheese lower in protein is ideal

Limit: Yogurt

Yogurt is interesting because for some people it can actually help get rid of acne. The reason for this is the probiotics typically found in yogurt, including s. thermophilus, l.bulgaricus, l. acidophilus, bifidus, l. rhamnosus, and l. paracasei. While these probiotics are great, they come at a pretty significant cost. Yogurt is also high in lactose, casein, whey, and calcium, all of which contribute to acne. If you are going to use yogurt, try to stick to the following:

- Full-fat (low-fat yogurt usually has sugar & vegetable oils)
- Go with plain, non-flavored yogurt, and add raw honey or berries if you *need* to
- Greek yogurt is preferred – it's higher in probiotics and healthy fats

Limit: Whey Protein Powder

Yep, most protein powder counts as dairy too – whey is simply milk protein.

Due to the fact that whey protein powders contain large amounts of the dairy protein, whey, they should generally be avoided for clear skin as well. Despite not containing lactose or casein A1, whey by itself is enough to trigger symptoms of acne.

- One study found whey protein powder to trigger a larger amount of insulin than white bread[7]
- Another found that whey dramatically increased IGF-1[8]

In addition to this, many whey protein powders contain additives and sugars that can aggravate acne even more. If you are going to use whey, go with pasture-raised and choose only the highest quality. Overall, it's tough to find a protein powder that's ideal for clear skin. I would recommend sticking to real foods instead of protein powder if you can.

Unsafe: Ice Cream

Ice cream tastes amazing, but it comes at a huge cost. In addition to all the other negative aspects of dairy, like IGF-1, high amounts of lactose, and casein, ice cream will also trigger a huge insulin spike just from all the sugar that's added. What you get is a double-dose of hormonal trouble: insulin, IGF-1, and other hormones are triggered by both the dairy found in ice cream *and* the sugar.

Dairy buying guide

When it comes to dairy, the animal's diet and how it was raised makes a huge difference when it comes to hormones and nutrition.

If you are going to eat dairy, here are the elements you want to look for in dairy:

- Grass-fed and organic (fewer omega-6 fatty acids)
- Raw/unpasteurized (pasteurization kills all the good bacteria found in dairy and makes it less nutritious)
- Fermented/aged (can help decrease IGF-1 content)
- Full-fat (lower insulin response)
- Goat and sheep products are preferred (their genetic makeup is closer to humans, so there is a smaller likelihood of hormonal acne being triggered)

Nuts and Seeds

Many nuts and seeds are great choices for clear skin because they are typically low in carbohydrates and high in healthy fats, which make them unlikely to trigger insulin-driven acne. On the flip side, many nuts and seeds are likely to cause inflammation-driven acne due to a large amount of inflammation-causing omega-6 fatty acids. Furthermore, nut and seed intolerances are extremely common, and these can cause acne.

The key with nuts and seeds is two things: moderation and testing. Many nuts on this list (like brazil nuts) are great sources of hard-to-find nutrients, but also really high in antinutrients. Thus, you need to figure out which nuts and seeds work for you.

Safe: Macadamia nuts

Macadamia nuts are one of the single best foods you can eat for clear skin. They are low in omega-6 fatty acids, they're full of healthy, insulin-blunting monosaturated fats, and they contain very few antinutrients that could cause inflammation or intolerances. They aren't loaded with nutrients, but sensitivities to macadamia nuts are extremely uncommon and they're among some of the easiest nuts to digest.

Safe: Hazelnuts

Hazelnuts are a great source of skin-friendly nutrients including vitamin E, manganese, and magnesium. They're low-carb and pretty high in protein too. They have less omega-6 than almonds and can be soaked to decrease phytic acid content. Intolerances to hazelnuts are less common than almonds, which makes them a slightly better choice for acne-prone skin.

Safe: Chestnuts

Unlike most of the other nuts here, chestnuts are low in protein and fat. Instead, they have plenty of carbs and very few nutrients. While they're not likely to give you any major issues apart from potentially increasing blood sugar (still, not a ton of carbs per serving, so nut a huge concern), they're not going to give you any real health benefits either. They're likely safe for your skin, but won't be doing it any favors.

Safe: Pistachios

Not only do pistachios taste good, but they're a good source of vitamin K, loaded with prebiotics, and relatively low in antinutrients too. All in all, they're not as nutritionally dense as almonds or as low in inflammatory fatty acids as macadamia nuts, but with moderate consumption, they shouldn't cause any issues in most individuals. They are a little higher in carbs, so if you're sensitive to insulin-driven acne, this could be an issue.

Test it: Almonds

On paper, almonds seem like an acne-fighting nutritional powerhouse. They're one of the best sources of vitamin E on the planet, loaded with prebiotics, and high in magnesium. Vitamin E is crucial for proper antioxidant functioning that leads to clear skin, and almonds appear to be one of the best ways to get them. So what's the problem? Almonds are also high in antinutrients and inflammatory fatty acids which cause acne.

If you eat too many almonds, it's likely you'll find yourself breaking out. Intolerances to almonds are also *extremely* common. Soaking almonds can help decrease the amount of antinutrients they contain, though.

The same goes for almond butter, almond flour, etc., of course.

Test it: Cashews

Cashews have a decently high level of omega-6 fats, they're higher in carbs, and have a good amount of phytic acid. Cashews are a high FODMAP food, so they may cause issues in certain individuals. Intolerances to cashews are also relatively common, but if you can tolerate them, they're not an awful choice either. Cashews are also high in oxalates, so if you're attempting to avoid oxalates for any reason, I recommend cutting out cashews.

Limit: Brazil Nuts

Brazil nuts are an interesting food – they're pretty massive in size, indigenous to South America, and highly coveted by many South American tribes. Nutritionally speaking they're one of the only good sources of selenium on the planet, but they're also extremely high in antinutrients, especially omega-6 fatty acids and phytic acid. For this reason, if you can and do eat brazil nuts, stick to a handful or so per day.

Limit: Pecans

With very few carbs, a decent amount of protein and only moderate levels of phytic acid, pecans look decent on paper. Where we run into issues is the omega-6 fat content. Just a handful of pecans can throw your whole omega ratio out of the window and lead to acne-causing inflammation. Moderation is key here.

Test it: Sunflower seeds

Sunflower seeds are a great source of one of the most important nutrients for proper skin hydrating and antioxidant functioning – vitamin E. Unfortunately, sunflower seeds are also very high in inflammation-causing omega-6 fatty acids. That's why it's critical to test sunflower seeds for yourself, and whenever possible, go unroasted or dry roasted.

Test it: Flaxseed, Chia Seeds

While you certainly want to avoid flaxseed and chia *oil*, flaxseed and chia themselves are actually relatively low in omega-6 fatty acids when compared to other nuts and seeds. Again, you'll want to test them, but because most of their polyunsaturated fats are in the form of omega-3, they shouldn't be as problematic as other seeds.

Limit: Pumpkin Seeds, Sesame Seeds

Pumpkin and sesame seeds are both extremely high in omega-6 fatty acids with relatively few nutritional benefits for your skin. If you can, opt for healthier nuts or seeds or consume in moderation.

Unsafe: Peanuts

Although peanuts aren't technically considered a nut, they're often consumed like one. Despite being delicious, peanuts are one of the single worst foods that acne-prone individuals could eat. Not only are they loaded with phytic acid and lectins that can severely damage your digestive system, but they have an abysmal omega-fatty acid profile.

Do yourself a favor and opt for healthier nuts like macadamias or almonds whenever you can. This is especially true for peanut butter, which often contains inflammation-triggering vegetable oils – stick to almond butter if you have to, or macadamia butter if you can find it.

Note: Always buy unroasted or dry roasted nuts

Nuts are almost always roasted with canola oil, or some other vegetable/seed oil high in omega-6 fatty acid, so it's paramount to get unroasted or dry roasted nuts. Even if you're eating a safe, low-omega-6 nut, like a macadamia nut, if it's roasted in canola oil you'll be eating tons of oxidized, inflammatory fatty acids anyway, making it considerably more likely to trigger inflammatory acne. Whenever you can, opt for dry roasted or raw nuts and seeds.

Finally, make sure you always check the nutrition label, not just for inflammatory oils that may have been used for roasting but also for added sugar. A lot of nuts and seeds might have a flavoring or "honey glaze" that's really just sugar. While nuts and seeds are great sources of healthy fats, if you're eating sweetened nuts then your body may trigger an acne-causing insulin spike.

Meat & Eggs

Meat is generally an extremely safe food for acne. Meat, by virtue of the fact that it's animal-based, contains very few potential antinutrients that could trigger inflammation or intolerance issues. Plants have to develop anti-nutrients to avoid being eaten. Animals, on the other hand, run, flee, and fight – hence, they're generally some of the easiest foods to digest due to a lack of antinutrients.

That doesn't mean that some meats can't cause issues, but in general, meat is a great choice because it's low in carbs and high in fats, meaning it avoids not just inflammatory acne but also insulin-driven hormonal acne. You don't have to eat meat to get clear skin, but most people find it helpful. Where you need to be careful with meat is potential intolerance to histamine or nitrates, and omega-6 intake. Overall, though, most meat is a great choice, especially ruminants (cattle, sheep, goat, elk, bison, etc.), herbivorous mammals that ferment plant-based foods. They're easier to digest and loaded with nutrients.

Safe: Lamb, Goat, Sheep

It might be hard to get your hands on goat or sheep, but lamb is a common meat that's available pretty easily and is hands-down one of the best choices of food for acne-prone skin. Lamb is almost exclusively sold grass-fed, which means fewer omega-6s and more anti-inflammatory omega-3s. Lamb is also a zinc powerhouse, which makes it one of the only solid dietary sources of zinc outside of shellfish and oysters. Overall, it's a great choice.

Safe: Bison, Elk, Venison

Bison is in the same camp as lamb – a little hard to come by, but almost always free-range and organic. No reason not to indulge in it.

The same goes for elk and venison – there simply isn't "factory farmed" game meat out there.

Safe: Beef

Beef is a generally extremely safe choice for acne. While grass-fed beef is often ideal as it contains more omega-3s and fewer omega-6s, Dr. Shawn Baker found that the difference between factory-farmed beef and grass-fed beef was a lot smaller than we'd previously considered. For most people the difference will be negligible. Beef triggers a relatively small insulin spike, and being a ruminant is easy to digest. Obviously go for grass-fed if you can, but don't worry about it if you can't afford it or find it.

It depends: Poultry (chicken, turkey, etc.)

Poultry is kind of the odd meat-based food that may not be the based for your skin – it doesn't have a lot of nutrients, and they're often very high in inflammation-causing omega-6 fatty acids. Chicken or turkey skin, in particular, is extremely high in omega-6, which can cause inflammation-driven acne. While factory-farmed chicken and turkey contains a lot more omega-6 than free-range chicken and turkey, even free-range poultry is relatively high in it. For these reasons, I'd say opt for safer sources if you can, but don't fret about it too much – these are still low-carb, easy to digest foods.

It depends: Pork

Pork is interesting because in certain cases, it's actually been shown to trigger massive insulin spikes despite having no carbs[31]. There is a lot of speculation as to why this is – in some studies, cured pork performs better than uncured pork in this regard, and pork prepared in apple cider vinegar and salt showed beneficial effects. Personally, I can do other meats just fine, but for whatever reason I can't do pork. I can quite literally feel the insane insulin effect as I sprawl out for a post-bacon nap. Test it out – if you don't experience this, I say go for it, but just be wary.

It depends: Eggs

On one hand, eggs are an acne-clearing powerhouse. They're loaded with retinol vitamin A, vitamin D, vitamin E, riboflavin, biotin, and zinc, all some of the most important nutrients for clear skin. On the other hand, they're one of the single most common intolerances out there and depending on the type of egg you buy they might even be loaded with inflammation-causing omega-6 fatty acids. The culprit of these issues is surprisingly egg *whites*.

Egg yolks get a bad reputation for their cholesterol content (which again, is due to a debunked fad that "cholesterol is bad"), but in reality, the part of the egg that the vast majority of people are sensitive to are egg whites. Egg yolks contain all the nutrients, including biotin and riboflavin, two nutrients that are crucial for beating fungal acne and dermatitis.

Egg whites are high in protein, but also high in antinutrients.

The purpose of the egg white is to protect the egg yolk, in a sense, and so it's not surprising that many people have egg white intolerance (plus egg whites contain compounds that bind to biotin and prevent it from being absorbed, which can impact hair and skin health). If you tolerate egg whites just fine, then don't worry about it, but if you eat a lot of eggs and struggle with acne you might want to try eating just the egg yolks.

Furthermore, factory-farmed eggs contain several times the amount of omega-6 fatty acids, and a fraction of the healthy nutrients. If you can, opt for pasture-raised eggs. The yolks should be vibrant, large, and bright orange, not yellow. The shell should require a decent amount of pressure to crack them. Overall, eggs are one of the first foods I think you should test – but if you *can* tolerate them, I think they're an amazing choice.

Liver and Other Organ Meats: Nutrient-Dense Foods Loaded with Vitamin A

I wanted to make a separate section for liver and organ meats and leave them until the end for a reason – they are some of the few *true* nutrient-dense, acne-fighting foods out there.

Throughout this section, you've probably noticed a familiar trend – plant-based foods are great, but many of them contain antinutrients that prevent your body from absorbing certain nutrients, or they have nutrients but in the wrong form (e.g.: beta carotene vitamin A, ALA comega-3, etc.).

So, it begs the question, for tens of thousands of years of human history, where were humans getting many of these essential nutrients, like vitamin A, zinc, and omega-3 from? Liver and organ meats are the answer.

Take vitamin A, for instance. Vitamin A is absolutely critical for fighting acne. In fact, it is easily one of the most important nutrients, and helps combat pretty much every root cause of acne:

- Reduces the size of sebaceous gland, which is responsible for producing the oil that can lead to acne[32]
- Improves wound healing (can help heal acne scars faster)[33]
- Acts as an antioxidant that protects the skin against free radicals
- Helps prevent dead skin cells from clogging pores and protects the skin from UV damage[34]
- Reduces inflammation[35]
- May play a role in decreasing the risk of thyroid disorders[36]

Liver is the single best source of retinol (usable) vitamin A on the planet. It's *loaded* with vitamin A, so much so that no other food really comes close. Other organ meats contain similar benefits which are difficult for any plant-based foods to match.

The moral of the story here is simple – try your best to incorporate organ meats, especially liver, into your diet. Beef, lamb, bison, elk, and goat organs are ideal, but pork, turkey, and chicken organs are also viable sources. If you can't stand the taste or can't find organ meats, there are good, desiccated organ supplements that can help you get the benefits of organ meats. The downside is that they're quite expensive. See the Supplements chapter for more information.

Side-note: getting vitamin A on a plant-based diet

While the absolute best way to increase your vitamin A intake is by eating organ meats (or taking desiccated organ supplements), if you're sticking to a plant-based diet you can still make sure your body is getting plenty of vitamin A by doing a few things:

- Sweet potatoes are the plant-based king of bioavailable

vitamin A. They have much more vitamin A than other vegetables or roots and are a generally healthy food overall, if you can tolerate a moderate amount of carbohydrates and plant-based foods.
- Cook or sauté your vegetables with a healthy fat (ghee, avocado oil, olive oil, etc.) or sprinkle some olive oil on your salad. Vitamin A is a fat-soluble vitamin and eating it with fat can drastically increase nutrient absorption of vitamin A[37].
- Lightly cook or steam your vegetables. For the most part, intense cooking or baking will break down nutrients found in vegetables, but cooking vegetables (especially in a healthy fat!) can also make them easier to absorb. Generally speaking, gently sautéing, baking, or steaming is the way to go if you want more nutrients without sacrificing flavor.[38]

Fish and seafood

Fish and seafood are some of the safest foods you could possibly eat for acne. They contain practically no carbohydrates, which makes them safe for avoiding acne-causing insulin spikes. They also don't contain plant-based antinutrients that can damage the gut, making them generally easy to digest and gut friendly. Furthermore, many fish contain acne-fighting nutrients, like zinc, omega-3, and vitamin D to help fight off inflammatory and hormonal acne.

Safe: Wild-caught salmon

Wild-caught salmon is practically the ultimate acne-fighting superfood. It's rich in omega-3 fatty acids that help fight inflammatory acne, low in inflammation-causing omega-6 fatty acids, and is one of the best sources of the astaxanthin, an extremely potent antioxidant that protects the skin. As an added bonus, it's rich in vitamin D, selenium, vitamin B6, iodine, and biotin too (crucial for combatting fungal acne).

Wild-caught salmon is a nutritional powerhouse with very few drawbacks. On the flip side, farmed salmon is an entirely different story. It has upwards of 6 times more inflammatory omega-6 fatty acids than wild-caught salmon, and most farmed salmon is riddled with antibiotics that can damage the digestive system.

Overall, stick with wild-caught salmon whenever you can, and if you can't afford wild-caught salmon, opt for a more affordable alternative like sardines.

Safe: Sardines and Anchovies

Sardines and anchovies are loaded with omega-3 fatty acids, are very low in omega-6 fatty acids, and are an excellent source of vitamin D and selenium. Plus, the only sardines (and most anchovies) you can buy are wild-caught. With the added benefit of being low in mercury, there's really no reason *not* to add sardines and anchovies to your arsenal.

Safe: Mackerel

Mackerel is the king of omega-3s, with more per serving than any other fish. It's also low in omega-6 and high in retinol vitamin A, vitamin D, selenium, magnesium, and zinc, all of which are great for our skin and health. Again, you ideally want to opt for wild-caught mackerel, as otherwise you'll be offsetting the effects of the omega-3s with plenty of omega-6 fatty acids.

Safe: Oysters

Two words: zinc powerhouse. Oysters are one of the single best sources of zinc on the planet, which can help fight inflammatory *and* hormonal acne. Oysters also have a little bit of omega-3 and solid amounts of vitamin A, vitamin E, and selenium. Obviously be careful of allergies or intolerances, but if you can handle them, then oysters are a great choice.

Safe: Squid

Squid, as long as it's not fried (calamari), offers many of the same benefits of oysters, but to a lesser degree. What you want to avoid is fried squid, or calamari. The breading alone can cause an insulin spike that triggers hormonal acne and digestive issues that could cause inflammatory acne.

Safe: Tuna

Tuna is an okay source of omega-3s and has a relatively small amount of omega-6, as well as having a few other nutrients like selenium, vitamin D, iodine, and potassium. The downside to tuna is that they're usually high in mercury, especially if farmed. Again, not a huge issue as long as long as you consume tuna in moderation.

Safe: Trout

Trout is a little bit higher in omega-6 fatty acids than other fish, but not by a large degree. It's a good source of vitamin D, selenium, and some omega-3s. Like tuna, it's high in mercury, and without a ton of acne-fighting nutrients, there's not a huge reason to add trout to your diet.

Safe: Walleye, Mahi, Mahi, and Trout

Walleye, mahi-mahi, and trout all fall into about the same camp. They don't have a ton of acne-fighting nutrients outside of selenium, but there's also no reason they should make your acne worse.

Safe: Clams and Mussels

Clams and mussels are good sources of a handful of vitamins and minerals necessary for clear skin, including manganese, magnesium, selenium, and vitamin A. They're also pretty good sources of omega-3 fatty acids too (with very little omega-6). Like the fish above, they're a generally safe choice for acne-prone skin without any massive health benefits.

Safe: Lobster and Crab

Both lobster and crab are very high in zinc and good sources of selenium and copper. They're both also extremely low in omega-6 and have a few omega-3s of their own. The downside is that they're high in vitamin B12, which has been shown to make acne worse, and that intolerance to them seems more common than to other types of fish. If you can tolerate them, they're a great choice.

Unsafe: Tilapia

Tilapia is not only one of the worst fish you could eat for acne, but one of the worst foods for your health overall. They're very low in useful nutrients, and very high in harmful chemicals, dangerous bacteria, and toxins that can affect our skin and our health.

Farmed tilapia is commonly fed animal feces, which can cause toxicity and sickness. It was found that the vast majority of tilapia imported from China was fed animal feces[39] which can lead to dangerous bacterial consequences.

On top of animal feces being in your tilapia, harmful, banned chemicals usually make their way into Chinese tilapia sold around the world[40]. Tilapia is one of the only fish you should avoid for clear skin.

Vegetables

Vegetables are generally extremely safe and nutritious foods for clear skin. Most vegetables are very low in carbs and high in fiber, which makes them ideal for preventing insulin-related acne. With that being said, some vegetables are high in certain antinutrients that may cause issues in some individuals, which is why testing is critical.

This section is going to be a little bit different, simply because vegetables as a whole are some of the safest foods you can possibly eat for acne. The vast majority of people can enjoy a plethora of vegetables without worrying about acne.

Still, for some, vegetables high in FODMAPs, oxalates, or other antinutrients can cause specific issues. That's why, instead of going over each vegetable individually, we're going to go over groups of vegetables that might be problematic depending on your situation.

Furthermore, how you prepare your vegetables can greatly impact the amount of antinutrients, so we'll cover how to cook vegetables as well.

If a particular intolerance or sensitivity doesn't apply to you, then assume that the vegetable is safe for clear skin or refer to the Protocols section for which vegetables to avoid for your exact situation.

Nightshades

Nightshades, including tomatoes, white potatoes, eggplant,

okra, peppers, gooseberries, pepino melons, paprika, and cayenne, are a family of fruits and vegetables that contain a chemical called solanine. Solanine is generally safe to consume, and most people are unaffected by solanine; however, many individuals with autoimmune or inflammatory conditions, like acne, report nightshade intolerance. For this reason, you may want to try cutting out nightshades for a period of time if you struggle with inflammatory acne.

High-FODMAP vegetables

FODMAPs are carbohydrates that *some* individuals have a challenging time digesting. Individuals report inflammation and digestive issues upon eating them, and many people find that eating a low-FODMAP diet may help with acne.

- Artichoke
- Asparagus
- Beets
- Broccoli
- Brussels sprouts
- Cabbage
- Cauliflower
- Eggplant
- Fennel
- Garlic
- Kale
- Leek
- Mushrooms
- Okra
- Onion
- Peas
- Shallots
- Spring onion

- Snow peas
- Sugar snap peas

It is not necessary (and possibly not ideal, even) to limit high-FODMAP foods; however, if you find yourself sensitive to them, you may want to avoid these high-FODMAP vegetables in order to gauge intolerances for a period of time.

Vegetables high in oxalates

Oxalates are another antinutrient found in some vegetables that can cause issues for *some* people. Oxalates are created by the fungus aspergillus and yeast candida, both of which can cause digestive issues that may be related to acne. The following vegetables are high in oxalates:

- Raw kale
- Rhubarb
- Raw spinach
- Raw chard
- Beets

Just like many other antinutrients, the high-oxalate content of many vegetables can be reduced by simply cooking or steaming these vegetables.

Vegetables to buy which should be organic

While there is no scientifically proven link between the consumption of conventional or organic food and acne, there are some vegetables that experts almost unanimously agree should be bought from organic sources due to an otherwise high chemical and pesticide content. These include:

- Spinach
- Kale

- Celery
- Potatoes
- Hot peppers

Cooking vegetables for optimal nutrition

Most vegetables that *can* be cooked, *should* be cooked, very lightly. The reason for this is simple – while cooking vegetables will destroy *some* of the water-soluble nutrients, the vast majority of fat-soluble nutrients (like vitamin A) found in vegetables hold up well under cooking, while most of the antinutrients (including FODMAPs, oxalates, and phytic acid) that can cause acne are diminished greatly.

Basically, while cooking your vegetables will make them a little less nutritious when it comes to water-soluble vitamins, it'll also make them a *lot* easier to digest, which for acne is our main goal.

Furthermore, cooking vegetables the *right* way can actually increase nutrient absorption. One study showed that consuming fat with beta carotene, the type of vitamin A found in vegetables, could increase bioavailability substantially[41]. That's why it's generally best to cook your vegetables as lightly as possible, with steaming, light sautéing with a skin-safe fat, or lightly roasting with a skin-safe fat like olive or avocado oil.

Avoid searing or baking at high temperatures, as you'll end up destroying even the fat-soluble nutrients with harsher cooking methods.

Fruits

Just like vegetables, *most* fruits, in their raw form and in reasonable quantities, are very safe for acne-prone skin. In fact, unlike vegetables, fruits rarely contain many antinutrients as they don't require as much protection thanks to their skins, shells, and innate protection mechanisms.

For the reasons above, we're going to use the same approach as vegetables and simply go over certain categories of fruit that might give you troubles depending on your own current dietary situation and lifestyle factors.

The key with fruit is to make sure that *if* you have insulin sensitivity or insulin-driven acne, that you're careful when it comes to eating fruit that's too high in sugar. Most fruits have a lot of sugar, but also a lot of fiber to offset the insulin spike, making them considerably safer. Opting for lower-sugar, higher-fiber fruits is the best strategy when it comes to fruit.

Safe: Avocados and olives

Both avocados and olives are extremely high in healthy fats and extremely low in sugar, which means that unlike other fruits, they won't trigger an acne-causing insulin spike even if you happen to overindulge in them.

Olives are also extremely high in vitamin E, which happens to be a crucial, acne-fighting nutrient that helps protect the skin from oxidization and damage that can lead to acne.

Some people are sensitive to both these fruits, and avocados are relatively high in FODMAPs and histamine (again, only a problem if you find yourself sensitive to them after, something we'll talk about more later), but overall, they're one of the best snacks you can have for clear skin.

Don't eat *too much* high-sugar, high glycemic index fruit

Some fruits can be pretty high in sugar and low in fiber, which means they'll elicit a large insulin response from the body that can cause acne. Below is a table with data regarding GI of some of the most common fruits:

FRUITS	GI
Apple	39
Banana, ripe	62
Dates, dried	42
Grapefruit	25
Grapes	59
Orange	40
Peach	42
Pear	38
Prunes, pitted	29
Raisins	64
Watermelon	72

Watermelons have a very high GI, while raisins, grapes, and bananas also have relatively high GIs. You probably don't have to avoid these fruits by any means, but just be aware that overindulging in them may cause issues.

High FODMAP fruit

Just like our list of vegetables, many fruits that are generally safe to eat may be problematic if you have FODMAP sensitivity issues. These fruits include:

- Apples
- Apricot
- Avocado
- Ripe bananas
- Blackberries
- Boysenberries
- Cherries

- Dates
- Figs
- Mango
- Nectarine
- Peach
- Pear
- Permission
- Plum
- Prune
- Watermelon
- Dried Fruit
- Fruit Juice

Avoid Fruit Juice (see "Drinks" For More Details)

On paper, fruit might look problematic for acne because of the sugar content – but the thing is, when you eat a fruit, there's plenty of fiber mixed in, along with dozens of other nutrients and compounds that help blunt the insulin effect and aid in the digestion of the fruit. When you drink fruit juice, you essentially strip the fruit of everything that makes it nutritious – especially the fiber.

The fiber found in fruit is absolutely necessary for it to be considered safe for your skin – fruit juice, which is almost always fiber-free, is basically just overpriced sugar water. It's very likely to spike your insulin levels which can contribute to acne, and the nutrients in fruit juice are few and far between.

Long story short, just avoid fruit juice if you want clear skin.

Nightshades

As discussed in the "Vegetables" and "Starches & Grains"

sections, nightshades are a family of fruits and vegetables that may cause inflammation and other autoimmune issues (including acne) in certain individuals. If you think you have a nightshade intolerance or sensitivity, you may want to consider cutting these fruits out for a period of time:

- Tomatoes
- Goji berries
- Ground cherries

Fruit to buy which should be organic

Like vegetables, there are certain fruits that are more susceptible to carrying potentially damaging and harmful chemicals if not bought from organic sources. While we do not have evidence that this is linked to acne, it is generally recommended that you buy the following fruit as organic:

- Strawberries
- Tomatoes
- Nectarines
- Apples
- Grapes
- Peaches
- Cherries
- Pears

Drinks

By far the safest and best drink when it comes to acne is simple: water! Aside from moderate amounts of fluoride found in most tap water across the United States, there is absolutely nothing about water that can damage your skin.

While you may have heard that green tea is the key to clear skin, or that herbal remedies are crucial, the simple fact of the matter is that while green tea *can* be a great choice for individuals who tolerate it, we all react differently to the caffeine, fluoride, and other compounds found in something like tea.

That's why, when in doubt, I highly recommend going with water – there isn't a single person on the planet who's intolerant to it. With that being said, some drinks are better than others – we'll go over them below.

Safe: Water

Safe and ideal. If you can, get water that's free or low in fluoride (e.g. spring water/reverse osmosis filter/alkaline filter), but I wouldn't worry about this too much. Slightly fluorinated water is still safer than pretty much anything else out there, and oftentimes it's not worth the hassle of trying to find anything different.

Limit: Coconut Water

Coconut water is easy to digest and rarely problematic when it comes to autoimmune conditions or things like acne. The only problem with coconut water is that it will spike insulin levels due to the sugar contained in it. It's not the worst thing in the world for most people, but I wouldn't recommend it on a regular basis.

Test it: Kombucha

I'm separating kombucha from traditional tea because it's really quite different – by undergoing a fermentation process, kombucha typically has less caffeine than other tea and added probiotics. While this sounds great, we know relatively little about the gut microbiome, and while some people find that it helps with digestive issues and acne, other find that it hurts (likely due to the moderate amount of sugar in kombucha). Definitely give it a go, but don't be surprised if it's not for you.

Unsafe: Soda

This one is pretty obvious - in addition to being high in caffeine which can disrupt sleep and increase your stress response, soda is loaded with sugar, which triggers an insulin response from the body and can lead to hormonal acne. Even diet soda is often loaded with compounds and chemicals that mimic sugar in the body and trigger an insulin response. It's much safer to go with sparkling water, as even diet soda can trigger acne-causing hormones and is loaded with chemicals.

Unsafe: Fruit juice

Fruit juice, whether it's apple, orange, grape, or some other type of juice, takes everything that is healthy and beneficial about fruits and throws them out completely. Without the naturally occurring fiber found in whole fruit, fruit juice is essentially sugar - it'll trigger a significant insulin spike that can cause acne and won't carry nearly the same benefits as eating a whole fruit with regards to antioxidants and fiber.

Unsafe: Anything with added sugar

There are tons of energy drinks, sports drinks, and other concoctions out there that I simply won't have the space to cover at length – the key thing to look for when buying these drinks is added sugar content. A single sport drink oftentimes has as much sugar as your favorite soda but is marketed as a "fruit drink" or an "electrolyte drink" that's supposed to be healthy for you. Unless you are a world-class athlete, you don't need 40 grams of sugar for your workout (and likely still don't).

Similarly, in the absence of fiber, your body doesn't care if the sugar is coming from a plant-based, "healthy" source – you're still going to have a significant insulin spike that can lead to acne.

When in doubt, go with water.

Unsafe: Milk (Cow, Sheep, Goat, etc.)

See "Dairy".

Safe: Coconut Milk

Coconut milk is by far the safest dairy milk alternative for clear skin. Very, very few people have coconut intolerances, which makes it safe when it comes to digestive issues that arise from antinutrients. It's low in sugar and carbs, and overall an extremely safe choice - just make sure you get sugar-free coconut milk.

Safe: Macadamia Milk

Macadamia milk, much like coconut milk, is an extremely safe choice when it comes to dairy-free milk substitutes for clear skin.

The reason for this is simple: macadamia nuts themselves are an extremely safe, easy to digest, and low-carb food that is unlikely to trigger inflammatory or hormonal acne. They're rich in healthy monosaturated fats and very low in inflammation-causing omega-6 fatty acids (unlike a lot of other dairy-free milk substitutes).

Test It: Almond Milk & Cashew Milk

Almond milk and cashew milk are decent choices, but both are relatively high in omega-6 fatty acids, and nut allergies are common. On the plus side, they contain prebiotics that may aid digestion and are low-carb options that are unlikely to trigger insulin-driven acne. In any case, I would highly recommend going with coconut milk, but if you can tolerate them, they're not awful choices either in moderation.

Unsafe: Oat Milk

Oat milk has many of the same issues as oats themselves – high in lectins and antinutrients, and it triggers a pretty decent insulin spike due to the carb content. I'd opt for one of the choices above before choosing oat milk, but I also don't think it's going to kill most people. I'd say for most individuals it's still a better choice than dairy milk, but not ideal by any means.

Unsafe: Hemp, Flaxseed

Hemp and flaxseed milk are *loaded* with omega-6 fatty acids that can trigger inflammation. Plus, just like hemp and flaxseed, some people have intolerances to them, making them poor choices. Overall, opt for coconut, macadamia, almond, or cashew milk.

Unsafe: Soy Milk

Soy is a well-known hormone disrupter and extremely high in phytic acid and potent lectins. While it's a good low-carb alternative milk, it's simply not worth the price that your digestive system will pay.

Important: Issues with Tea and Coffee

Below we'll go over several different types of tea and coffee, but it's important to note the two largest downsides to many types of tea and coffee before we begin: fluoride and caffeine.

Fluoride is a neurotoxin that has a whole host of negative effects on our body, but the chief one that we're worried about is how it effects our thyroid health. The thyroid is a gland near the throat that influences a wide array of hormonal functions in the body. It's one of the most important organs when it comes to having proper energy levels, stress responses, mood, and body temperature.

Unfortunately, fluoride significantly influences how much thyroid hormone your body produces, and can contribute to something called hypothyroidism, which is a condition frequently associated with autoimmune disorders like acne, especially in women[42].

Fluoride and acne have such a strong tie that researcher Melissa Gallico wrote an entire book just on fluoride and its relation to acne. Many teas are extremely high in fluoride, which also means that they could be causing thyroid-related acne. Coffee does not contain significant amounts of fluoride. See the Thyroid Protocol chapter for a detailed look at how to beat thyroid-driven acne.

Secondly, tea and coffee are very high in caffeine, which in addition to being dehydrating to the body (and thus the skin), stimulates an extremely high stress response in the body. Chronic stress can lead to a plethora of issues, but for our purposes, the most important is the impact it has on proper digestion, gut microbiome diversity, and sleep. All of these factors can make us more susceptible to acne.

Overall, if you *can* cut out coffee and tea, I'd recommend it. Do I think it's necessary for most people? Absolutely not. If you get a lot of joy and value out of a cup of tea or coffee, I think it's better to find ways to clean up your diet in other ways rather than cutting out genuine sources of happiness in your life.

Without further ado, lets jump into the specifics of several types of tea and finally coffee.

Test it: Black Tea

Black tea is the most popular form of tea and the type with the most proven benefits, alongside green tea. It has actually been shown to increase insulin sensitivity, which can help prevent hormonal acne. There are also some studies showing that the prebiotics can help increase gut microbiome diversity. Finally, it contains antioxidants that can help protect the skin from free radicals.

The downsides are pretty straightforward – black tea is high in caffeine and pretty acidic, which can disrupt the digestive system, and also has pretty high levels of fluoride.

Safe (Generally): Green Tea

Without a doubt, the largest benefit of green tea is that it's loaded with skin-clearing antioxidants. Green tea generally has more antioxidants than any other type of tea. In particular, it's loaded with EGCG (151mg / cup), an antioxidant that can help decrease levels of acne-causing hormones and sebum oil, prevent inflammation, and protect the skin from sun damage and acne-causing free radicals.

Green tea contains 35-45mg of caffeine per cup, which is about average when it comes to caffeinated teas. Still, it's about three times less caffeine than a cup of coffee, and, like black tea, was shown to have only a moderate effect on stress hormones when compared to other forms of caffeine[43].

Unfortunately, green tea is also very high in fluoride, containing roughly 1.6mg per liter. That's about the same as two cups of tap water in the United States. Again, you'll want to see if you're sensitive to fluoride or not. You can minimize fluoride content by going with tea that was grown either in Japan or the Pacific Northwest instead of China.

Safe: White Tea

White tea is the least processed tea and also arguably the safest caffeinated tea for acne-prone skin. It has the lowest caffeine content of any caffeinated tea, very high levels of ECGC antioxidants, and low levels of fluoride and heavy metals. White tea isn't studied in medical or nutritional literature nearly as much as black or green tea, so our knowledge of its potential benefits is a bit more limited.

Test it: Oolong Tea

Oolong tea is mainly consumed in China and requires a much longer and more intensive brewing process than other teas. Oolong tea is right between green tea and black tea when it comes to caffeine content, with 37 – 55mg per cup. Again, that's still less than half the amount of caffeine in a cup of coffee. It has more antioxidants (EGCG) than black tea (81.58mg/cup) and shows pretty much the same benefits for acne that other teas containing ECGC show: lower inflammation, less insulin, protection against UV and free radical damage. Oolong tea has about as much fluoride as your typical black or green tea (1.32 mg/liter), so on that front, it may be problematic for individuals with thyroid issues.

Furthermore, if you struggle with eczema, oolong tea might be a unique solution. One study found that 63% of patients with eczema noticed an improvement in their skin after one month of consuming a liter of oolong tea per day.

Limit: Coffee

In my personal experience of running the GoodGlow blog, I've seen ten to twenty times more people have problems with coffee than with tea.

I think that there are a few reasons for this:

- Tea is higher in antioxidants
- Tea usually has a compound called L-Theanine in it, which helps promote a healthy stress response and can offset some of the effects of caffeine
- Tea has less caffeine than coffee (oftentimes by a significant amount)
- Most tea is less acidic than coffee, which makes it easier to digest
- Tea intolerance seems to be far less common than coffee intolerance

Again, it's hard to find hard data against coffee, simply because most of the studies analyzing coffee are either done by coffee producers and manufacturers, or coffee alternatives (soda companies) looking to skew research in favor of coffee alternatives, although one study did find that caffeine (without L-theanine, found in tea) can essentially double the body's natural stress response[44].

All I can really say here is that if you struggle with acne and drink coffee, I recommend first switching from coffee to white or green tea, and then, if problems persist, cutting out tea altogether. I know that's tough to swallow, but you might find that coffee, or possibly caffeine in general, was the trigger that was holding you back from clear skin.

You don't need to make the shift all at once – start by switching to half green/white tea and half coffee for a week, then three quarters green/white tea and one quarter coffee the next, and finally completely over to green/white tea on week 3. The same protocol can be used to wean yourself off tea, simply replacing caffeinated tea with herbal tea.

Safe: Herbal tea

Herbal tea isn't really "tea" in the traditional sense. While all the other types of tea come from the same plant, camellia sinensis, herbal tea is a collection of herbs, spices, and dried plants that have a similar effect to tea when steeped in hot water. That doesn't mean that herbal tea isn't beneficial for acne – in a sense, it's actually the safest "tea" for acne-prone skin because it doesn't have any caffeine. It's also extremely low in fluoride (0.02 – 0.09mg/Liter).

Common ingredients in herbal tea, like turmeric, spearmint, peppermint, lemon, ginger, and rose, have pretty powerful effects, ranging from improving digestive health to lowering inflammation and insulin levels. They might not single-handedly cure your acne, but they can be a great substitute for sugary drinks or even regular tea if you're sensitive to caffeine.

The following herbal tea ingredients are unique to acne:

- Spearmint and peppermint tea have been shown to decrease levels of DHT, a male sex hormone that can cause oily, acne-prone skin (lowering DHT isn't necessary for clear skin and is oftentimes unideal for men, but can be effective for some individuals)
- Turmeric is a great anti-inflammatory compound that can reduce the effects of inflammatory acne
- Ginger has been shown to improve digestion, which can play a role in nutrient absorption, insulin, and food sensitivities related to acne
- Cinnamon has been shown to increase insulin sensitivity, which as we know is great for acne-prone skin

Alcohol

Can you drink and still have clear skin? Yes, of course! While alcohol is generally problematic when it comes to your skin due to its dehydrating properties, ability to disrupt the gut microbiome, and its effect on insulin resistance, what's often most problematic about alcohol isn't necessarily the alcohol itself, but the rest of the beverage.

Tequila isn't the absolute worst thing in the world, but if you're drinking it in a sugary concoction, it's a whole lot worse. No alcohol is better than any alcohol when it comes to your skin, but that's also a pretty unrealistic standard to set – most adults enjoy an alcoholic beverage from time-to-time, and knowing which ones are best for your skin may come in handy. For this reason, here's a quick breakdown of alcoholic beverages.

Safest (but Still Not Great!): Tequila, Gin, Whiskey, Vodka, Rum

These are about as pure and safe as you can get when it comes to alcohol for acne-prone skin. In their pure forms, these hard liquors are low-sugar, low-carb, low-antinutrient drinks. All in all, your body will have to deal with the alcohol and not much else.

But what about mixed drinks with these hard liquors in them? Well, that's where you can run into issues. Always avoid mixed drinks with anything other than sparkling water. I know, I know, it's boring, but your skin will thank you for it.

Limit: Wine

Wine probably seems like one of the safer choices for alcohol, but many wines are actually a nightmare for acne. Commercial wines are typically loaded with pesticides, additives, and coloring agents that can trigger inflammation and sensitivity issues in certain individuals. Sweet wines contain tons of sugar that can cause inflammation-driven acne, and many wines are also high in yeast which can worsen issues like candida.

Still, if you choose the right type of wine, you can minimize all of these downsides. Try to find *natural* wine, not just organic or low-carb wine. Natural wine contains no unnecessary sulfites, coloring, additivities, or pesticides that can contribute to acne, and they never have added sugar or sweeteners.

Okay: Champagne and Sparkling Wine

All real, authentic champagne comes from a specific region in France that utilizes lower-toxin farming than most other types of alcohol. In addition, authentic champagne must meet pretty high safety standards to be labeled "champagne".

When it comes to other sparkling wine, including prosecco, there's usually a bit more sugar and generally fewer rules and regulations regarding the quality of the grapes. Just like regular wine, you need to be careful about what types of sparkling wine you buy. It's usually even harder to find natural sparkling wines than it is regular wines, so proceed with caution.

Pretty Good: Hard Cider

Hard cider is actually pretty decent for you compared to beer – it's gluten-free, grain-free, and usually very low in yeast and antinutrients that prevent you from absorbing zinc, a crucial nutrient for clear skin. Not to mention hard cider tastes amazing – but that great taste comes at a cost.

The problem with hard cider is that it's almost always high in sugar. A single bottle of your average hard cider can have over

30g of sugar. As we know, sugar is a nightmare for acne. If you can find a dryer, less sweet hard cider, then you're looking at a pretty skin-friendly drink. Unfortunately, most ciders sold in the US are really sweet and loaded with sugar.

Unsafe: Sweetened Mixed Drinks

Moscow mules, dry martinis, and (unsweetened!) margaritas; what could go wrong? Actually, in the case of these unsweetened mixed drinks, not a whole lot. At their core, these mixed drinks are sugar-free, skin-friendly hard liquors like tequila, gin, and vodka with some citrus and water.

What about piña coladas, long islands, rum and coke, or fruity margaritas? That's where you run into problems.

All of these drinks have an insane amount of sugar, not to mention a ton of calories too. They're almost guaranteed to spike the acne-causing hormone, insulin, and the added ingredients can trigger inflammation or food sensitivities too.

Unsafe: Beer

Most beer is loaded with carbs, which can trigger a cascade of hormones that cause acne. A single can of regular beer has over 12g of carbs on average. While light beer has about half the carbs, it still doesn't escape the other drawbacks of beer and acne.

Beer contains gluten, a common trigger ingredient that can damage the gut and, in certain individuals, lead to inflammatory acne. It also contains small amounts of phytic acid, an antinutrient that blocks zinc, one of the most important nutrients for clear skin, from being absorbed.

On top of that, most beer includes its fair share of yeast and mold bacteria, which again can trigger inflammation and lead to nasty yeast infections (like candida) that can make it much more difficult to properly digest food and absorb crucial nutrients. As someone who's dealt with a yeast infection and could only get rid of it through fasting, trust me - it's not fun.

If you're going to drink beer, light beer is your best bet. It's lower in sugar and carbs.

Fats and oils

Most nut, vegetable, and seed oils are high in inflammation-causing omega-6 that can trigger acne. Furthermore, these oils typically oxidize at very low cooking temperatures, which makes them even more likely to cause damage. The key is to use fats that are low in omega-6, stable at high temperatures, and loaded with healthy saturated and monosaturated fat, including extra-virgin olive oil, tallow, ghee, coconut oil, avocado oil, and macadamia nut oil.

Safe: Coconut oil

In addition to containing lauric acid and MTCs that boost energy, coconut oil is anti-inflammatory, anti-bacterial, and anti-fungal. Best of all, coconut oil is low in omega-6 fatty acids that spur inflammation and can cause acne to form. There is some evidence that the capric acid found in coconut oil might also be useful for fending off and recovering from digestive issues like small-intestinal bacterial overgrowth.

It has a relatively low smoke point so you won't want to use it for high-heat cooking, but overall, it's a pretty good choice.

Safe: MCT oil

MCT oil is just coconut oil with the non-MCT (medium-chain

triglycerides) removed. There is no reason for MCT to be any less safe than coconut oil for your skin, although cooking with MCT oil is usually pretty rare.

Safe: Grass-fed ghee/grass-fed butter

We've covered both these options in the dairy sections already, so for a more detailed look at these fats, see that section. Ghee is ideal because butter contains trace amounts of lactose, casein, and whey, which can cause issues in certain individuals, whereas ghee is pure butterfat. Ghee has a very high smoke point, making it ideal for high-heat cooking.

Safe: Olive oil

Olive oil is packed with antioxidants, safe for vegetarians and vegans and fairly low in inflammatory fatty acids. There's very little to be worried about with olive oil. Despite having a higher amount of omega-6 fatty acids than the other fats on this list, olive oil contains anti-inflammatory antioxidants that help counteract the omega-6 content, and it's nowhere near as high in omega-6 as your typical vegetable oil.

Try to go with organic, extra-virgin olive oil over regular olive oil when you can. It has fewer free radicals than regular olive oil and more antioxidants. Also, always try and get olive oil in a tinted bottle and store it in a cool, dark location – olive oil is very sensitive to light, and the omega-6 fatty acids can oxidize if not properly stored, making them a bombshell for your skin.

Safe: Avocado oil

Avocado oil has a very high smoke point (400 degrees), which makes it an ideal plant-based alternative to olive oil for high heat cooking. Similarly, like olive oil, it is extremely high in vitamin E, a crucial antioxidant for healthy, hydrated skin. It also contains the anti-inflammatory antioxidant oleic acid.

Safe: Beef tallow

Tallow doesn't have any insanely positive health benefits like olive oil or ghee butter, but there's nothing really dangerous about it either. With an extremely low amount of omega-6s and a high smoke temp, it's ideal for high-heat cooking. With considerably less omega-6s than lard, it's really the ideal animal fat alongside ghee.

Safe: Duck fat, other animal fats

Most other animal fats (see section below for information on lard) are safe for consumption. It's relatively rare to see low-quality duck, goat, or sheep fat or tallow being sold because they're generally a delicacy. Again, go for high-quality brands when you can, but I wouldn't worry too much about that.

Limit: Cacao Butter

Cacao butter is rich in monosaturated fat and has no carbs. It's plant-based and has a very high smoke point. It has a relatively high amount of omega-6 so you might want to consider limiting it, but nowhere near as much as oils like canola or other vegetable oils. Overall, I'd say avocado oil or olive oil are better choices, but if you're going for a plant-based butter substitute this is a good choice.

It Depends: Lard

Lard from pasture-raised pigs is actually pretty healthy – it's (relatively) low in omega-6 fatty acids and has a high smoke point, which means it's a lot more stable than many other vegetable oils.

With that being said, conventional lard is extremely high in omega-6 fatty acids due to the lower quality diet and lifestyle of factory-farmed swine, which can trigger inflammatory acne.

Limit: Canola oil

Canola oil isn't quite as high as the other vegetable oils on this list in omega-6 fatty acids, but it's still up there. Given that there are many other, safer, plant-based options out there, like avocado, macadamia, or olive oil, I'd recommend limiting or avoiding canola oil whenever you can.

Limit: Nut Oils (except macadamia nut oil)

The problem with nut oils (like almond oil) is that they're very high in inflammation-causing omega-6. So, even though almond oil is probably a safer choice than soybean oil, for instance, due to the high vitamin E content and overall better nutritional profile, it's still not a great choice. Macadamia nut oil is a good exception, as it has very little omega-6.

Unsafe: Vegetable & seed oils (list below)

This includes soybean oil, wheat germ oil, corn oil, sesame oil, peanut oil, cottonseed oil, grapeseed oil, flaxseed oil, sunflower oil, margarine, shortening.

The reason you want to avoid these vegetable oils is simple – they're loaded with inflammation-causing omega-6 fatty acids. Although it might *look* like some of these oils have enough omega-3s to counteract it, like flaxseed oil, the unfortunate reality is that the omega-3 found in these oils is ALA omega-3, which has to be converted to EPA and DHA omega-3 before it can be used by the body (and the body is *very* inefficient at doing this). So, basically, all you're left with is extremely sensitive omega-6 fatty acids which can trigger inflammation.

Spices & Herbs

Spices and herbs are *generally* safe, but again, they're one of those weird areas where some people have a hard time tolerating certain spices. I'm going to label most of the following spices and herbs as "safe" but bear in mind you should test them.

Safe: Sea Salt/Pink Himalayan Salt

Not really a "spice" per se, but sea salt or pink Himalayan salt are both great, safe choices for your skin. There is absolutely no evidence to suggest that sodium plays any role in the formation of acne, and the "low-sodium" fad of the 80s has since been repeatedly debunked.

Safe: Cinnamon

Cinnamon has been shown to have a pretty profound impact on blunting insulin, making it great for avoiding hormonal acne. On the flip side, some individuals claim that cinnamon contributes to atopic dermatitis. There are no studies to back this up, but just something to keep in mind if you struggle with fungal acne, perioral dermatitis, or dandruff.

Safe: Oregano

Oregano is anti-fungal and anti-bacterial, which can actually help improve your gut microbiome and possibly fight off acne.

Safe: Turmeric

Turmeric is a *potent* anti-inflammatory. It doesn't taste great, but I'd highly recommend adding it to your diet if you are looking for an extra boost in beating inflammation-driven acne.

Safe: Cilantro, parsley, rosemary, lavender, thyme, cloves, basil

No issues here. No massive anti-inflammatory or insulin-blunting effects either, but no need to worry about them.

It depends: Paprika, garlic, black pepper, onion, mustard/mustard seeds

All of these spices and herbs have something in common – they're common intolerants and triggers of inflammation. If you've ever sneezed after eating pepper, or maybe your sinuses have clogged up, this is part of the reason why. If you can tolerate them, great, but if you have the option to cut them out, I'd recommend it.

Unsafe: Sugar, Coconut Sugar, Cane Sugar, Brown Sugar, most artificial sweeteners

Sugar is sugar. Sugar spikes insulin levels, destroys the gut microbiome, and even damages your teeth. Don't be fooled by "healthy" sugar alternatives, like coconut sugar or cane sugar. Your body doesn't care where the sugar came from, and neither should you when you're making purchasing decisions.

Avoid foods with added sugar, period. This includes *most* artificial sweeteners (see below), as they also illicit a sugar-like insulin response, despite having no sugar on a nutrition label. They're essentially the same thing.

It Depends: Stevia & Xylitol

I separate stevia and xylitol here from other sweeteners because studies show that their impact on insulin production is considerably milder than other sweeteners and sugars. For this reason, I'm putting them in the "It Depends" category. If you're putting sugar in your coffee and tea and just *need* some sweetener, make the switch to xylitol or stevia. Ideally you should use neither, but it's not the end of the world either.

Other Foods

These are some common misfits – they might fit into more than one food group or just be unique within their respective groups.

Unsafe: Milk chocolate

Milk chocolate contains dairy, sugar, and many allergens that are likely to trigger acne. It's a generally poor choice for acne-prone skin. Go for high-cacao dark chocolate if you need to satisfy the chocolate craving.

Limit: Dark chocolate

Dark chocolate on paper looks okay. It's loaded with antioxidants, and it's extremely high in fat and (generally) low in carbs, making it an ideal low-insulin snack.

There are a few issues with dark chocolate, though:

- It contains caffeine, so if you're sensitive to caffeine it can be a problem
- It's *extremely* high in phytic acid, an antinutrient that can worsen acne
- It's very high in oxalates
- A lot of people have a hard time tolerating dark chocolate

While extremely high cacao dark chocolate is superior, one study found that even 99% dark chocolate (practically no sugar) made acne worse.[45] If you can tolerate dark chocolate, it's a great choice. For the rest of us, try to avoid it, and if you must have it, go for a high-cacao (85% or more) dark chocolate.

It Depends: Protein Powder

Generally speaking, I'd recommend avoiding protein powder in favor of whole foods. But, if you must go with a protein powder, there are some things to look out for. Most plant-based protein powders contain pea protein. While many people can tolerate it just fine, others have a really challenging time with it. Be sure to test it.

When it comes to animal-based protein powders, collagen is king. Whey or casein protein powders are dairy, which leads to frequent irritation and sensitivity that can exacerbate inflammatory acne. Collagen protein (or beef gelatin) doesn't have that same issue and may actually help with skin repair and wound healing.

Still, no matter what protein powder you go with, make sure you avoid anything with added sugars or flavors.

It depends: Honey

Honey is a double-edged sword.

On one hand, our body knows *exactly* what to do with honey – we've been eating it for centuries and we've evolved alongside honey, eating it *infrequently* and seasonally. Honey is easy to digest, and there are actually certain health benefits to eating honey. It's anti-bacterial and anti-fungal, which can help certain individuals struggling with digestive issues. It can even help with seasonal allergies and sleep.

On the other hand, honey is *still* an insulin-spiking sugar substitute. It's not something you should be eating a ton of, and when you do eat it, make sure it's unpasteurized, raw, and preferably local – this will ensure you get all the health benefits while minimizing the downsides. When baking or cooking, if you *need* a sugar substitute, I'd recommend going with either honey or stevia.

"But Wait, What About…"

Phew, that was quite the list, huh?

You might be thinking to yourself, "This is great, but what about pizza, or my favorite turkey sandwich, or a gluten-free pie recipe I found online, are those okay too?"

The previous several chapters are meant to be a reference for *whole food ingredients* that make up other foods. It's simply unrealistic to go through each food (pizza, hamburgers, pie) in full detail – rather, use the previous chapters to analyze a food from a holistic perspective.

Burgers, for instance, contain beef – which is usually good! And lettuce, too, which oftentimes isn't problematic. But they also have bread (a no-go) and cheese, too. If a food contains something that you should avoid, or limit, it doesn't matter how many great, "nutritious" ingredients it has, it falls into the "unsafe" camp.

On the flip side, let's say your burger is on a coconut flour bun and dairy-free. It's low carb, and you season it with some salt. Any problematic ingredients here? Nope? Then you're probably in the clear.

As you can see, going over *every* food would be impossible – what counts as a "burger"? Should we include dairy-free, gluten-free pizza in our definition of "pizza"? That's why, in the next chapter, we'll go over some basics of analyzing various foods to quickly figure out whether or not it's likely to trigger acne based on the principles we just covered. Within seconds, you'll be able to navigate a supermarket like a pro.

Chapter 7: How to Analyze Any Food for Clear Skin

In the previous chapter, I tried to include information on as many foods as I realistically could. These common foods should account for 90%+ of the ingredients found in common foods. Still, in the USDA food and drink database there are *thousands* of foods listed. It's simply not feasible to list all of them here (nor would you want to read over a list of thousands of foods).

For that reason, I'm going to include a short section on how you can analyze just about any food and determine the impact it might have on your skin. Here is *exactly* what to look for on a nutritional label and ingredients list for clear skin.

1. What do the macros look like?

Macronutrients are carbohydrates, fats, and protein. This is one of the first things you should look at if you deal with hormonal, insulin-driven acne. There's no magic number to look for here, as the key thing isn't necessarily the total amount of carbs or fat, but rather the ratio between the macronutrients.

For instance:

- Foods that are primarily carbs generally trigger a higher insulin response.
- Foods that are primarily protein generally trigger a moderate to low insulin response.
- Foods that are primarily fat generally trigger a low insulin response.

See which macronutrient contributes to the calorie count the most. You can use free apps like Chronometer or even just look at the nutrition label.

While there's no specific amount of carbs per day that is ideal for everyone, *most* people generally find it helpful to stick to less than 50-75 *net* carbs for acne (more on that below).

2. Check sugar (and fiber)

Alright, so let's say a food is relatively high in carbs. Does that mean you should *definitely* avoid it?

Not necessarily.

Always check to see how much *sugar* a food has. Anything over 10g *without* fiber is generally problematic, and anything with more than a gram or two of "added sugar" is something you definitely want to avoid.

On the flip side, also check the amount of fiber in a food. Fiber doesn't trigger a blood sugar response – in fact, it helps slow down our insulin spikes. So, while a food might have a decent amount of carbs, if it has a lot of fiber you'll be good to go (assuming you can tolerate it).

As an example, an avocado has 12g of carbs, which isn't insignificant, but 10g of those 12g are fiber. So, basically, it only has 2g of "net" carbs. You can always subtract the amount of fiber from total carbohydrates to get a better idea of the insulin impact. Fiber is why *real* fruits are so much healthier than fruit juices.

3. Check the ingredients for vegetable oils

If a food has practically any fat, you're going to want to check the ingredients label for vegetable oils. The amount of omega-3 and omega-6 isn't required to be listed on nutrition labels (even though they should be), so you're going to have to do some guesswork here.

Look out for these ingredients, and if possible, avoid foods that contain them: soybean oil, wheat germ oil, corn oil, sesame oil, peanut oil, cottonseed oil, grapeseed oil, flaxseed oil, sunflower oil, margarine, shortening, and canola oil.

4. Look out for other additives and hidden ingredients

There are also a few hidden ingredients that can trigger acne if you're not careful.

These include sweeteners, like:

- Any mention of "syrup" (e.g. corn syrup, maple syrup, high-fructose corn syrup, agave syrup, golden syrup)
- Cane sugar/cane juice crystals
- Molasses
- Coconut sugar
- Date sugar
- Fruit juice/fruit juice concentrate
- Dextrin
- Dextrose
- Glucose
- Maltose
- Maltodextrin
- Fructose
- Xylose
- Sorghum

Sugar is sugar. While coconut sugar is marginally better for you, it's still not something you should indulge in. Xylitol and stevia should be avoided, if possible, but studies show that they have fewer negative effects in general and are *better* but still not *ideal* substitutes.

And wheat and grain-based ingredients:

- Any mention of "Wheat" (e.g. wheat bran, wheat germ, wheatgrass, whole wheat etc.)
- Any mention of "Flour" (e.g. bread, cake, enriched flour, pastry)
- Any mention of "Starch" (e.g. gelatinized starch, modified starch, modified food starch, and vegetable starch)
- Any mention of "Gluten" (many products will say whether or not it's gluten-free)
- Any mention of "Cereal" (e.g. cereal grains, cereal extract)

The following names are also used for wheat:

- "Fu"
- "Seitan"
- "Farina"
- "Bran"
- "Matzo"
- "Germ"

Any mention of "Corn":

- Corn syrup (especially high-fructose corn syrup)
- Corn sweeteners
- Corn starch
- Corn oil
- Maize

Any mention of other grains:

- Any mention of "Oats"
- Any mention of "Barley"
- Quinoa
- Kernels

- Farrow
- Kasha
- Bulgur

5. **Rules of thumb for Grocery Shopping**

Don't want to spend time looking at every single nutrition label? Don't worry, here are five "rules of thumb" to stick to when grocery shopping:

1. Avoid "low-fat" or "reduced-fat" products – I've said it before, and I'll say it again – fat isn't bad for you and it doesn't make you fat. Low-fat products contain more sugar, more industrial fats, and more artificial ingredients that spike insulin and trigger inflammation.

2. Stick to the outside perimeter of the grocery store and buy whole foods – most grocery stores have a similar layout – fresh and whole foods along the edges, and processed, artificial foods in the middle and down the aisles. You want to be where the whole, unprocessed food is.

3. The shorter the ingredients list, the better – while this isn't always true, it's a pretty good rule of thumb. If you buy a "Paleo-friendly" power bar with 36 ingredients in it, odds are some of them aren't great for your skin. Skip it and buy whole foods instead.

4. Don't sweat it if you can't afford organic – If you can afford organic, wild-caught, pasture-raised, or wild-caught food, that's great! But as a whole (with the notable exception of factory-farmed fish), eating *conventional* whole foods is far better than eating *organic* processed foods. Overall, there's a relatively small difference between the nutritional content of organic and conventional food, so don't sweat the small stuff.

5. Frozen vegetables are often better – Ideally, you're buying fresh vegetables at your local farmer's market, but in reality this isn't always an option. Quick-frozen vegetables are often "fresher" than fresh vegetables that have been sitting on the shelves for days on end. They're a lot cheaper too – Trader Joe's has organic frozen spinach for $2/pound.

Section III: Meal Timing & Fasting

Meal Timing & Fasting

This is going to be relatively short section, but I think it's an extremely important one – in fact, perhaps *the* most important section *depending* on who you are. Fasting, even intermittently (skipping a meal or two) can have an *enormous* impact on inflammation, insulin sensitivity, and the gut microbiome. Yup, that's *all* the root causes of acne.

For this reason, some people subscribe to the notion that *when* and *how often* you eat is just as important, and sometimes *more* important, than *what* you eat. Personally, intermittent fasting was the missing puzzle piece for me – despite eating very cleanly, I was eating far *too often* and not giving my digestive system enough time to rest. Incorporating intermittent fasting actually allowed me to eat some foods that I'd previously had a hard time digesting, and overall made a huge difference to my skin and my health.

Now, before we even begin, I really, really feel like I need to add this disclaimer again: talk to a health professional *before* incorporating intermittent or prolonged fasting into your clear skin strategy. I am *not* a doctor. This is *not* medical advice. You may have some underlying conditions or factors that could put you at risk when fasting. While many doctors and physicians are tentative about recommending fasting, there are a growing number of health professionals who are eager to adopt and implement intermittent fasting protocols for weight loss, autoimmune disease, and healing. It's worth seeking out these professionals who can help you plan to fast safely.

It's also worth noting that just like how different foods affect everyone differently, intermittent and prolonged fasting affects everyone uniquely. It might make a *huge* difference for some people (like myself). For others, it might actually make acne *worse*. There's a mountain of clinical research for the benefits of intermittent fasting on all the root causes of acne, but that doesn't change the fact that for a small minority of people, intermittent fasting can increase stress or cause the opposite effect. I'll do my best to outline who's at a higher risk for these sorts of issues throughout the chapter, but the key to answering this for yourself is to first speak with a healthcare professional and then to *test* several strategies for a period of time.

There is an acclamation process with any of these protocols where your body needs to adjust, so it's best to *ease* into these strategies rather than jumping in headfirst. I'll provide some information about what has worked for me and what clinical research seems to suggest in terms of adopting fasting successfully.

Chapter 8: Intermittent Fasting for Clear Skin

The basic idea of intermittent fasting is simple – eat all your food for the day during a short period of time, and don't eat (fast) for the rest of the time.

This usually means skipping a meal or two and having larger meals later in the day. It could be as simple as skipping breakfast or as extreme as having only one meal a day.

Intermittent fasting is not a diet – it isn't about what you eat, it's about when you eat. Intermittent fasting can be looked at as a pattern of eating, providing a framework for when you should and shouldn't eat throughout the day.

Does this mean you could eat pizza and spaghetti while intermittent fasting? Technically, yes – but it doesn't mean you *should* – that's why I recommend combining intermittent fasting with one of the other protocols I outline in this section for clear skin.

Intermittent fasting is a powerful tool that can amplify the results of your existing diet and help your body recover from dieting mistakes faster. It's not a license to eat acne-causing food and walk away untouched, but it can be an extremely effective asset for clear skin.

The health benefits of intermittent fasting are huge:

- Decreased risk of certain cancers[46]
- Improved learning and memory performance[47]

- Promotes cardiovascular health[48]
- Reduced blood sugar and increased insulin sensitivity[49]
- Increased stress tolerance
- Better sleep[50]
- Reduced inflammation[51]
- Increased life span & anti-aging[52]

The reason for these benefits is simple – the body, quite frankly, is not meant to eat as frequently as we make it. Anthropologic evidence suggests that for the vast majority of human history, we were not eating three square meals a day. We would have periods when we were either low or deprived of calories. The body is meant to go through periods like this – it's what triggers a process called autophagy, where old, damaged cells are used as fuel in the absence of food. Fasting, quite literally, triggers our body to start eating unhealthy cells. It is the only real "detoxification" method that we have.

With specific relation to acne, the benefits for fasting primarily come down to decreased insulin resistance, which prevents hormonal acne, and decreased markers of inflammation. Insulin is really only released in large quantities when we eat food (some insulin can be released when we drink diet sodas, flavored waters, coffee, or tea too), so by limiting the number of times throughout the day we eat insulin, we give our body a chance to actually use the glycogen we have stored up in our cells instead of relying on blood sugar. On top of that, because intermittent fasting can be considered a state of acute, minor stress, the body releases anti-inflammatory cytokines during intermittent fasting. For this reason, it's important not to jump into a super intense intermittent fasting protocol if you deal with chronic stress.

Lastly, and probably most importantly, intermittent fasting gives our digestive system a much-needed break. Especially in the case of prolonged fasts, it allows the digestive system to heal and recover from the constant bombardment of food that we typically put into it.

How to incorporate intermittent fasting for clear skin

Again, just like every other protocol, the key here is to listen to your body and do what feels right. There are dozens of different types of intermittent and prolonged fasting, and here I'll go over several of the most common ones that can help with acne.

In this section, we'll focus on fasts that are less than 36 hours (and cover prolonged fasting in greater depth later).

16/8

This is the easiest and most popular method of intermittent fasting. You simply don't eat for 16 hours a day, and then eat for 8. Here's an example of what this might look like:

- 7:00am – Wake up, skip breakfast
- 11:00am – Start lunch
- 1:30pm – Snack #1
- 4:00pm – Snack #2
- 7:00pm – Finish dinner

The exact hours you fast don't technically matter. You could skip dinner if you wanted to or eat your first meal at 1pm.

It's worth noting that anecdotally it seems like people experience the most benefits eating only two meals a day and skipping snacks, as it gives the digestive system time to recover between meals.

16/8 is a really easy strategy to follow and skipping breakfast can actually add a huge amount of simplicity into your day.

Warrior Diet or 20/4

The "Warrior" diet is a very well-known program that involves fasting for 20 hours of the day and eating for 4. It's a simple technique that is a little more powerful than the 16/8, and it's something that I practice on occasion.

It's a lot more powerful than the 16/8, so if you're really looking to get some benefits from intermittent fasting, I think that this is a great balance of benefits and difficulty.

Here's a sample daily routine:

- Skip breakfast all day
- Begin eating period at 4:00pm
- Stop eating by 8:00pm

Most people eat two medium-sized meals during the four-hour window, but other folks will have a really long, large meal that they munch on over several hours. The eating window is small enough where there shouldn't be substantial benefits of choosing one approach over the other.

5:2 Method

The 5:2 Method is one of the more popular form of intermittent fasting and is ideal for individuals who would like to eat regularly on feeding days and keep fasting or meal timing to only two days a week. This method can work well for individuals who perhaps have to eat certain meals due to professional or social obligations.

This is a little bit trickier and requires you to restrict yourself to 500-600 calories two days a week (with at least one day in-between the fasts). For example:

- Monday – Eat normally
- Tuesday – Eat normally
- Wednesday – Eat 500-600 calories
- Thursday – Eat normally
- Friday – Eat normally
- Saturday – Eat 500-600 calories
- Sunday – Eat normally

Eat-Stop-Eat

This method involves a simple 24-hour no calorie fast once or twice a week. A 24-hour fast can be pretty tricky to pull off, so for many people this option isn't viable, but if you can muscle it, the benefits can be worth it.

An example schedule is below:

- Sunday: Eat normally
- Monday: Stop eating at 7:00pm
- Tuesday: Eat at 7:00pm
- Wednesday: Eat normally
- Thursday: Eat normally
- Friday: Stop eating at 6:00pm
- Saturday: Eat at 6:00pm

Many of the benefits that come from autophagy, the process where your body recycles old protein for energy, begins at 24 hours, so this can be a useful technique.

One-Meal-A-Day (OMAD)

OMAD is exactly what it sounds like – you eat one meal a day. It might sound crazy, but many experts argue this is likely the most similar eating pattern to our ancestors.

OMAD can simplify your day, jump-start weight loss, and

increase autophagy – a process where your cells recycle old, damaged proteins and replace them with new, healthy cells.

I currently eat one meal a day, not just for the acne-related benefits, but because over time it's naturally what my body has found most comfortable. I typically eat a very large, ~2,700 calorie meal (I'm generally very active) at the end of the day. Others opt to eat their one meal a day during the afternoon, while some even prefer the morning. While I've become accustomed to eating in the evenings, and find eating at other times to produce fatigue, it's all up to you *when* you eat your one meal.

If you do want to start doing OMAD, I recommend that you first begin with an easier pattern like the 16:8 or the Warrior Diet, and then ease into OMAD slowly (try a few Eat-Stop-Eats to get your body accustomed to it).

Chapter 9: Prolonged Fasting for Clear Skin

In addition to intermittent fasting, there is *prolonged* fasting, which is fasting for more than 24 hours. Prolonged fasting has gained a lot of interest lately due to influencers like Tim Ferriss who popularized his 3-day fasting protocol.

Prolonged fasting compounds on a lot of the benefits of intermittent fasting: it gives the digestive system a break, and it helps curb insulin resistance, decrease inflammation, and improve gut microbiome health[53]. In addition, prolonged fasting has two unique outcomes that typically don't occur when intermittent fasting: deep healing of autoimmune disorders and autophagy.

Studies have shown that prolonged, multi-day fasts (and fasting-mimicking diets, which we'll talk about shortly) have a profound and rapid effect on autoimmune conditions[54]. Individuals have found relief from acne, eczema, dermatitis, and psoriasis with prolonged fasting.

On top of that, prolonged fasting leads to something called autophagy, which is basically the process of your body recycling old, damaged cells. Because this is a cellular mechanism, it affects just about every organ and part of the body, giving you a full-body health boost that'll carry over to your skin. On top of that, many people experience extremely rapid and pronounced healing of old wounds and scars after completing a prolonged fast – this *could* help with acne scars. I've personally seen benefits related to acne scars after completing 6-day fasts.

Basically, prolonged fasts can supercharge your intermittent fasting goals, but should *only be done* by experienced fasters and under medical supervision. Again, I am not a doctor, and this is not medical advice – prolonged fasts *can* be dangerous; a lot more dangerous than intermittent fasting, at least, if done improperly. Fainting is far more common, for instance.

Furthermore, if you're underweight, or close to being underweight, you should likely avoid prolonged fasting.

There are several different and beneficial ways to complete a prolonged fast.

Prolonged Water Fasts

A water fast (no food or beverages besides water) is arguably the most beneficial way to complete prolonged fasts, but it's also quite challenging and daunting for many. We'll cover this in further detail in the "What Breaks a Fast" section.

A common question that arises is, "How long should I fast?" There are no studies around the impact of prolonged fasting specifically on acne, so instead I'll summarize the findings related to prolonged fasting and autoimmune disorders, inflammation, and insulin resistance:

- 24-36 hours: Autophagy, the process of old, damaged cells being recycled, begins at about 24 hours, so this is really the minimum length of time for a prolonged fast to be more effective than an intermittent fast
- 3 days: Powerful effects on the immune system, autophagy, insulin resistance, and inflammation – a perfectly adequate amount of time for a prolonged fast
- 7 days: Even more pronounced effects, wound healing results may begin - however, only safe for individuals in the moderate BMI range

- More than 7 days: Deep healing and extreme results for autoimmune disorders, but also potentially more dangerous

This is *not* a recommendation about how long you should fast. Again, this should all be discussed with a healthcare professional.

Fast-Mimicking Diet (FMD)

Because of the potential dangers that come with water fasting (and the generally negative or shy sentiment around it from healthcare professionals), it may be helpful to consult your doctor about the fast-mimicking diet (FMD) instead of the prolonged water fasting.

This protocol is pretty new, and honestly probably my favorite method here – I'm doing a FMD round right now as I write this book.

The fast-mimicking diet is exactly what it sounds like – it's a diet that *tricks* your body into thinking it's fasting. In simple terms, it's a period of caloric restriction in which you eat foods that avoid triggering a non-fasting bodily state, followed by refeeding.

The goal of the fast-mimicking diet was to allow people to reap many of the benefits of fasting without the extreme nature of pure water fasting. Studies show that it has many benefits related to key markers of adult acne – insulin resistance and inflammation chief among them[55].

There are "official" FMD kits with prepackaged foods and such, but honestly, I think that's just overpriced and gimmicky.

The easiest, and in my opinion, best way to do the fast-mimicking diet is simply to eat between 600 and 800 calories of high-quality fat per day, for 3-5 days. 5 days is ideal (and where most of the research-based benefits come in), but 3 is great too.

My fast-mimicking diet looks like this:

- Day 1: Cauliflower rice sprinkled with olive oil, and a large avocado
- Day 2: Avocado and a handful of macadamia nuts
- Day 3: Two handfuls of almonds, handful of macadamia nuts
- Day 4: Two large avocados
- Day 5: Coconut flakes, handful of macadamia nuts, cauliflower sprinkled with olive oil

The key is to avoid protein intake and focus on easily digestible foods, as protein is the primary mechanism for signaling pathways in the body that put us in a fasted state.

While the official FMD doesn't advocate for a high-fat meal plan (they recommend 45% carbs, 45% fat, 10% protein), if you want the most benefits for acne, high-fat is the way to go, especially if you can stick to skin-safe high-fat foods like avocados, olive oil, ghee, macadamia nuts, almonds (if you can tolerate them), and coconut, etc.

Again, you're not going to get *all* the benefits of a prolonged water fast, but in my opinion, it may be worth it as you're also not taking all the risks that come with water-only fasting.

Fat Fasting

Fat fasting is another form of fasting that has gained a lot of popularity lately.

Basically, fat fasting is exactly what it sounds like – you consume only fats to avoid triggering the spike of insulin (from carbs) and trigger autophagy (triggered by protein). Fat fasting often involves eating a spoonful or two of coconut oil around mealtimes to avoid needing to eat, and limiting calories to around

400-600 for the day.

You can also do fat fasting intermittently by consuming "butter" or "fat" coffee or tea (just a zero-calorie beverage with a tablespoon or two of MCT oil, ghee, butter, or coconut oil) for breakfast and lunch and then eat a full meal at dinner. Although I don't recommend caffeinated beverages if you can avoid them, this idea of consuming a tablespoon or two of fat to make either intermittent or prolonged fasting easier can be a useful tool.

Again, you're not going to get all the same benefits as you would from water fasting, but for a lot of folks this is a manageable middle ground where they can continue to get some fuel from fat and maintain their daily caffeine intake. I personally prefer the fast-mimicking diet (and we have more research to back it up) but this is still a viable option, especially if you struggle with insulin-driven acne.

Chapter 10: Fasting for Clear Skin Best Practices

This chapter is going to address some of the biggest questions regarding fasting and how you can optimize your fasts for clear skin.

What "Breaks" a Fast?

A lot of people ask what "breaks" a fast. Can you drink diet soda? What about black coffee? How about putting a little cream in that coffee?

Some fasting purists insist that the only *true* fasting is water fasting – that drinking anything other than water breaks a fast (while other even believe that *dry* fasting is the only real fasting, something I do *not* recommend).

Personally, I think that this is a pretty silly question to ask, because everyone's goals with fasting are different and unique. The question instead should be, "What will prevent me from achieving the physiological effects that I'm looking for?"

For some folks who maybe struggle with insulin-driven acne, consuming black coffee with a teaspoon of MCT oil during a fast will have a minimal impact, as it has a negligible impact on insulin. On the other hand, if you're intolerant to coffee or sensitive to stress-driven acne caused by caffeine, black coffee, despite having zero calories, is a bad choice.

The safest, ideal way to go is water fasting – but that doesn't mean that you *have* to water fast, or even that you *should*. If you need that cup of green tea in the morning to get through the fast, it might be worth keeping it in your fast in order to get the ball rolling.

Here are some general rules of thumb when it comes to what "breaks" a fast, but again, there are people out there who have experienced massive results with "dirty" fasts consisting of several diet sodas a day. Do I recommend you go down this route? No, but it just goes to show that there is no one-size-fits all answer to the question of "what breaks a fast".

Instead, I'll outline some things you should avoid depending on your *goals* with fasting and what root causes of acne you think are at play for *your* body.

Healthy Fats

Consuming *pure, healthy* fats, like those we outlined in the first part of the Diet section, have a negligible effect on insulin levels. If your goal of intermittent fasting is *purely* insulin-related, then consuming coconut or MCT oil is not going to have a major impact. In fact, some tests show that MCT oil actually increases blood ketone levels, which can make fasting even easier.

MCT and coconut oil will trigger the digestive system, though. So if you're trying to have the purest fast possible, avoid them, but if you need something to get through the day, a spoonful of coconut oil, ghee, or MCT isn't a horrible option.

Tea & Coffee

This is a *huge* debate for a lot of people. Some studies show that green tea actually *increases* autophagy[56], the process in which old, damaged cells are recycled and used as fuel (crucial for healing, can play a role in acne scar healing as well).

On the other hand, it will trigger the digestive system, as coffee and tea, despite having zero calories, still contain prebiotics and other compounds. Furthermore, individuals have done blood glucose tests and found that coffee and tea can actually trigger a small increase in insulin production.

Lastly, for some people intermittent fasting can lead to stress, and the caffeine found in coffee and tea only exacerbates these issues. For these reasons I'd generally recommend avoiding coffee and tea if you can, but don't feel like this is necessary. I've done several 4-day fasts where I drink tea or coffee and have experienced amazing results, and oftentimes it can make the fast a lot easier to complete.

It's worth noting, though, that this only applies to *black* coffee and *unsweetened, plain* tea. Sugar will break your fast, and because cream is high in lactose, it'll also trigger a significant insulin spike. That goes for the vast majority of artificial sweeteners as well. If you just have to put something in your coffee or tea (trust me, I get it, I used to do the same), go for a small amount of ghee, coconut oil, MCT oil, or cinnamon.

Diet soda

Alright, I'm just going to flat out recommend that you avoid diet soda outright. While diet soda looks fine on a nutritional label (contains zero calories and no sugars), the artificial sweeteners found in diet soda have been shown to trigger insulin spikes regardless[57]. Some diet sodas containing stevia, for instance, might be slightly better in this regard, but along with all the other chemicals and irritants found in diet soda, it's just not worth it.

Fewer than 50 calories

A lot of people make the argument that anything fewer than 50 calories doesn't break a fast. I don't have much to add here, other than that if you want to get the absolute best results, I'd recommend avoiding even 50 calories, but if you *do* have 50 calories, make it a pure fat. Creamer, sugar, honey, and even 50 calories of protein powder will all have a larger insulin spike.

Vitamins, Supplements, and Pills

With the exception of electrolytes (which we'll talk about in just a second), there's really no reason to be taking supplements while fasting. The majority of nutrients require food to be eaten with them in order for the body to absorb them (that's why whole foods, not supplements, are the optimal source of nutrients). Some people say that multivitamins, supplements, or prescription medications will break a fast – there is no conclusive evidence to suggest this, but also little reason to be supplementing while fasting.

Apple Cider Vinegar

Again, it's the same story here as the other no/low-calorie beverages. Technically, this "breaks" your fast, because it's not water, but is it going to kill you? No. Will it make your fast significantly better, somehow? No. If it helps you get through the fast, go for it.

Bone Broth

This is another one that comes up quite often, but I think the answer is relatively straightforward – if you can avoid bone broth, that's ideal, but it's also a really powerful drink that can help you replenish electrolytes and act as a source of comfort. On the flip side, many people find that once you get rolling on a fast, you'll notice after the first day or two that you're not even hungry anymore – if you're drinking bone broth, you might never quite get to this point, constantly putting yourself in a survival state of hunger. That's because bone broth has a decent amount of protein, so it'll certainty trigger a minor insulin spike which can cause hunger. Testing and personal preference is key here.

Branch-chain amino acids (BCAAs)

A high intake of BCAAs has been shown to trigger the release of insulin and increase insulin resistance[58]. Ideal? No. The absolute worst thing you could have on a fast? No.

Fasting Supplements

I alluded to this point earlier, but the majority of supplements are worthless and counterproductive while fasting.

Supplements are a new invention in the overall scope of human existence. Most nutrients require fat, prebiotics, or other compounds found in food in order to be absorbed properly. Vitamin A, for instance, is absorbed in miniscule quantities when taken in the absence of dietary fat (like olive oil, for example), but is absorbed in much higher qualities alongside fat. In their natural forms, whole foods contain the necessary components for their nutrients to be absorbed. In supplement form, this simply isn't the case (with most supplements, at least).

When you're fasting, you'll inevitably not have the fiber, prebiotics, and fat necessary to make use of these supplements, so they're not worth taking. Some supplements, like gummy vitamins, even contain small amounts of sugar that'll make your fast less effective. In general, it's just worth avoiding them, with the exception of *electrolytes* - including sodium, potassium, magnesium, and more.

Dr. Rhonda Patrick has talked in extreme depth about the

importance of electrolytes while fasting, but the key message is that your body depletes electrolytes at an accelerated rate while fasting[59]. This can actually put you at risk of dehydration, fainting, increased stress, poor sleep, irritability, and more. By simply supplementing with a few electrolytes during fasting, namely sodium, potassium, and magnesium, you can avoid these issues while keeping your clean fast intact.

Any potassium supplement will do, and simple Himalayan pink or sea salt can be used for sodium. I prefer Thorne Research magnesium supplements, but any reputable brand will do (or you can use magnesium chloride).

Who Should Avoid Fasting

Fasting is an extremely powerful tool not just for better skin, but for better overall health. With that being said, some people should not fast, or are at a higher risk of experiencing downsides from fasting.

Pregnant women, for instance, should avoid prolonged fasting, and consider opting out of intermittent fasting and instead do whatever feels natural.

Children under 18 should avoid fasting as well.

Individuals who are underweight (or who have an eating disorder or anorexia) should also avoid prolonged and most forms of intermittent fasting. The general recommendation is that if you have a BMI of under 18.5, you should avoid fasting, and that if you have a BMI of under 20, you should avoid fasting for longer than 24 hours. To calculate your BMI, you can search for a free calculator from the National Heart, Lung, and Blood Institute online.

With that being said, an extremely common misconception is that intermittent fasting is *only* for weight loss. That is completely, entirely untrue. While intermittent fasting *can* (and often does) make it easier to lose weight, it isn't a surefire way to lose weight. In fact, when I *started* intermittent fasting, I was on the low end of the recommended BMI for fasting at about 145 pounds. I gained 20 pounds eating between one and two meals a day for two years. I know eating a single 3,000 calorie meal a day sounds nuts, but for some people this type of eating works better and gives the digestive system the break they need to actually absorb nutrients. Avoid fasting if you're extremely underweight, but bear in mind that it's a viable skin-clearing tactic for most people regardless of weight.

Lastly, if you suffer from chronic stress or anxiety, intermittent fasting probably isn't for you. Intermittent fasting elevates cortisol levels, which can be problematic if you already have high cortisol levels from stress.

Again, these are just a *few* examples of who should not fast. The key is to see a healthcare or wellness professional and develop a plan that works for you, and to test your plan in action and adjust accordingly.

Fasting is a great way to get back in touch with your biological needs, so use this as an opportunity to listen to your body.

Section IV – Lifestyle & Supplements

Lifestyle & Supplements

Before we start this section, let me get one thing straight: **diet is the number one factor in the battle for clear skin.**

If you're eating an acne-causing diet and trying to patch it up with supplements, it's simply not going to work. Supplements are not a replacement for good food. In fact, I generally recommend taking the *least* number of supplements possible for clear skin.

Why? Because if you *need* supplements, it means you might have some gaps in your diet. There is a *select handful* of nutrients that we simply can't get through food alone, or don't have access to (omega-3 from wild-caught fish, for instance). In these cases, supplements make sense - however, in most cases, they are expensive and unnecessary.

Furthermore, I don't want to downplay the importance of lifestyle factors like sleep, exercise, and stress management – all of these are great tools. But the emphasis of this book is on diet. To summarize decades of research on all of these factors is simply impossible, and what works for some people (cardio vs. weight training, for example) doesn't work for others. I'll highlight the general philosophy of a healthy lifestyle for clear skin here along with some potential starting places, but I will not be providing an exercise program or workout for clear skin.

Remember, **diet comes first**.

Chapter 11: Supplements for Clear Skin

Nutrients are meant to be absorbed through food. Vitamins, including vitamins A, E, K, and D, all require dietary *fat* to be properly absorbed. Many probiotics require prebiotics found in the fiber of various foods to take root and work. Antioxidant capsules have been shown to not perform as well as antioxidants found in tea[60].

Whenever possible, food-based nutrients are superior to supplement-based nutrients.

With that being said, by virtue of the fact that we live *radically* different lives than our ancestors did, some supplements are quite necessary in this day and age. Furthermore, there may be some nutrients that you personally can't get for financial reasons *or* due to dietary intolerances. Maybe you can't afford wild-caught seafood, or perhaps you're intolerant to shellfish so you can't find solid nutritional sources of zinc.

In these cases, supplements are a great option – the key is to use them to complement an already healthy diet, not cover up faults in an unhealthy one.

Vitamin A

Vitamin A is a fat-soluble vitamin stored in the liver. It's necessary for proper skin, eye, bone, and immune health. It helps alleviate acne by touching just about every possible root cause:

- Reduces the size of the sebaceous gland (produces oil that

clogs pores)
- Improves wound healing (can help heal acne scars faster)
- Acts as an antioxidant that protects the skin against free radicals
- Helps regulate the skin shedding process and ensures dead skin cells don't clog pores
- Reduces inflammation

Overall, there isn't a single vitamin that's more important for not just covering up the symptoms of acne, but truly *preventing it*. That's why drugs like Isotretinoin actually function using hyper-doses of vitamin A-like compounds to prevent and treat acne (with some nasty side-effects, which is why I recommend avoiding them).

Unfortunately, most of us aren't getting enough usable vitamin A to prevent acne. On paper, it might seem like we're getting tons of vitamin A, but really, we're eating a form of vitamin A that is inefficient for the body to actually utilize.

There are two types of vitamin A:

- Provitamin A (Carotenoids) – Found in vegetables and most supplements. Must be converted into retinol before it can be used by the body.
- Preformed vitamin A (Retinol) – Found in meat, seafood, and some dairy. Can be used by the body immediately.

There's nothing wrong with provitamin A; in fact, most of us consume plenty of it from vegetables alone, but this is an extremely inefficient form of vitamin A which later needs to be converted to retinol. Unfortunately, as little as 3% of all provitamin A you consume actually ends up being converted to *usable* vitamin A[61]. You can up those numbers by consuming healthy fats, like olive oil or coconut oil with your vegetables, but it's still not as beneficial as consuming preformed vitamin A.

This means that even if you're eating *tons* of kale or spinach, you might *still* be deficient in vitamin A.

So, where can you get *retinol* vitamin A? Unfortunately, the best sources are foods that most people eat relatively infrequently – organ meats, and in particular, liver.

In an ideal world you can get your vitamin A from an ounce or two of beef liver per week. But, because a lot of people don't have access to chicken, pork, beef, or lamb liver, I also recommend supplementing with retinol if you don't have an easy way to incorporate liver.

The best supplements, in this regard, are all food-based. Several brands offer desiccated beef liver supplements that are tasteless and loaded with grass-fed liver. The only downside is that they're relatively expensive.

Other vitamin A supplements will work if they are retinol-based rather than beta-carotene.

Vitamin D3

Vitamin D3 is one of the most important hormones in the body (yes, you read that right, vitamin D is a hormone). It's hard to think of an area of our health that vitamin D doesn't impact – from our mood to our immune system - it's a pretty important nutrient. Vitamin D is responsible for the expression of more than 1,000 genes. Sadly, upwards of a billion people worldwide are deficient in vitamin D[62].

Our ancestors would naturally get tons of vitamin D from being outside; however, in modern times, we're spending much more time indoors, covered up, or slathered in sunblock.

Deficiency in vitamin D is a real problem for acne – one study found that 95% of people with acne were deficient in vitamin D[63]. It's hard to understate the importance of vitamin D when it comes to acne.

- Can help prevent chronic inflammation and regulate the immune system
- Influences genes that ensure skin cells die, shed, and don't clog pores
- Increases the absorption & utilization of magnesium, phosphate, vitamin K2, and other nutrients
- Plays a role in insulin secretion.

Ideally, you'll be getting your vitamin D from the sun, as very few foods contain meaningful levels of vitamin D. Luckily, it doesn't take much - just 15 minutes a day of "unprotected" sun exposure can be enough to provide all the vitamin D3 you need. It's also worth noting that overdoing it isn't good for your skin either – your acne might look better after a day of sunbathing, but sunburn can dry out the *healthy* oil on the skin.

Furthermore, and I know this is going to sound crazy, but make sure you avoid wearing sunscreen when possible. Of course, if you're outside for hours on end it's probably a good idea, but bear in mind that our ancestors were outside for extremely long periods of time without sunscreen. Most sunscreens contain ingredients that are likely to exacerbate any existing skin issue, whether that's acne, dermatitis, or eczema. Go for physical protection from the sun – a hat, long-sleeved clothing, shade, etc., instead.

If you *must* use a sunscreen, zinc oxide-based sunscreens are considerably less likely to make you break out than other, comedogenic oil-based sunscreens or harsher spray-based sunscreens. Zinc oxide actually has natural anti-bacterial and anti-fungal properties, so while I wouldn't recommend slathering on zinc-based sunscreen on the daily it's a considerably safer choice for acne-prone skin.

If you *aren't* getting outside for *at least* 15 minutes a day near peak sunshine hours (11am-2pm), if you live in a northern climate, or have darker skin, supplementing with vitamin D3 is likely a good strategy.

Taking between 500 and 1,000 IU of a high-quality vitamin D3 per 25 pounds of bodyweight a day is a good starting place. If possible, consume vitamin D with a small amount of a skin-safe fat, like coconut oil. I live in a northern climate without much direct sun exposure, and supplement with about 5,000 IU of vitamin D3 per day.

Zinc

We have solid, concrete, scientific evidence that supplementing with zinc can help decrease acne. One study found that just by taking 30mg of a zinc a day, patients could decrease their acne by nearly 50% in less than 3 months[64]. Another found that after 12 weeks of treatment with zinc, the mean acne score for patients fell from 100% to 15%[65].

The reason for this is simple – like vitamin D3, zinc is crucial for *hundreds* of biological processes that create the proper conditions for clear skin:

- Assists in the absorption and transportation of vitamin A
- Acts as an antioxidant to protect against acne infections and UV radiation
- Zinc deficiency is linked to an increased risk of bacterial

infection
- Regulates apoptosis, the process of skin dying and shedding
- Protects the gut & improves intestinal healing
- Helps prevent insulin resistance
- Improves sleep quality and decreases stress

Despite all these benefits, most of us don't get *nearly* enough through our diet alone. It's estimated that upwards of 2 *billion* people are zinc deficient[66]. Furthermore, multiple studies show that individuals with acne and other skin conditions are more likely to be deficient in zinc.

A big reason for this is that there aren't many dietary sources of zinc which aren't also loaded with phytic acid. If you remember from the diet section, phytic acid is an anti-nutrient that binds to zinc and prevents our body from absorbing it. So even though foods like lentils are high in zinc on paper, if you're eating a diet high in lentils, you won't actually be *absorbing* much of that zinc.

So, unless you're eating animal-based sources of zinc, including oysters, lobster, or lamb on a regular basis, consider taking between 15 and 30mg of zinc picolinate per day, which is roughly the amount individuals took in the clinical trials mentioned above.

DHA & EPA Omega-3s

This book has been all about omega-3s and omega-6s, so I won't bore you with any more than the essentials here. Instead, we'll focus on why, even if you're eating plant-based foods that *seem* to be loaded with omega-3, like walnuts or hemp seeds, you're probably not getting the right *type* of omega-3s.

DHA and EPA omega-3 are two extremely important omega-3

fatty acids for proper brain function, immunity, and resisting inflammation. Study after study has shown that increasing your DHA and EPA omega-3 intake is one of the single best ways you can prevent inflammatory acne. DHA and EPA are found in fatty, wild-caught fish, including sardines, salmon, mackerel, anchovies, cod liver, etc.

ALA omega-3, on the other hand, has to be converted to DHA and EPA omega-3 before it can be used in the body. That's why foods like walnuts or hemp seeds, which seem to be loaded with omega-3, are really a trap – a fraction of that ALA omega-3 is actually used by the body (a lot like beta carotene and vitamin A) and you're left with a bunch of omega-6s.

For this reason, it's paramount to get your omega-3 through wild-caught, fatty fish. If you can't afford wild-caught fish or don't enjoy seafood, I recommend opting for the *right* omega-3 supplement. The wrong supplement can actually cause acne if you're not careful.

Omega-3 supplements come in a lot of varieties – you've got fish oil, cod liver oil, krill oil, algae oil, and various plant-based forms. The most important thing is to opt for an omega-3 supplement that's high in DHA and EPA omega-3, as opposed to ALA omega-3. ALA omega-3 has to be converted to DHA before it can be used as an anti-inflammatory.

As an extra precaution I prefer either krill or algae omega-3 supplements, as fish oil and cod liver oil supplements have been shown to go rancid very easily, which can cause more harm than good. Oxidized fatty acids can actually trigger an inflammatory response, and studies have shown that rancid fish oils are considerably more common than you'd imagine.

Again, eating fatty fish once or twice a week is the ideal

situation, but if you can't get your hands on wild-caught fish, 300mg of DHA & EPA per day is a good alternative.

Magnesium

Magnesium is a lot like vitamin D3 – it affects hundreds of different biological processes throughout the body, and very few of us get enough of it.

Magnesium has been shown to decrease insulin resistance (great for hormonal acne), lower inflammation (great for inflammatory acne), and help with anxiety, sleep, and chronic fatigue, all of which impact our overall health and skin.

Even if you're eating *tons* of leafy vegetables, you're probably deficient in magnesium. There's relatively little you can do to dramatically boost your dietary-driven magnesium intake. Modern farming practices and depleted soil make it nearly impossible to get enough magnesium through diet alone, which is why the majority of Americans are deficient in magnesium[67]. For this very reason, most people should consider supplementing with magnesium on a daily basis.

There are a lot of different types of magnesium out there – I prefer magnesium chloride, which comes in a spray and is easily absorbed by the body, but I also use a powder-based magnesium carbonate. Just make sure you check the ingredients label; a lot of magnesium powders contain added sugar.

Iodine

Iodine is a nutrient that most of us don't get enough of, by virtue of the fact that one of the only dietary sources of iodine is kelp or seaweed.

Iodine is important for acne for a simple reason – it is crucial for a properly functioning thyroid, and without it, the risk of hypothyroidism becomes considerably higher.

It balances out the effect of fluoride (in toothpaste, tea, water, etc.) and ensures that your thyroid can produce the hormones necessary to fight off acne. Rates of acne are considerably higher among individuals with thyroid issues (see Thyroid Protocol for more details).

While increasing your iodine intake is really only necessary for those with thyroid issues, iodine deficiency is rather widespread, and considering the link between thyroid disorders and acne, it's not a bad idea. It's not absolutely essential, like vitamin A, vitamin D, and zinc, but it's a good idea nonetheless.

The ideal form of iodine is from kelp powder or kelp/seaweed-sourced supplements in pill form. 150mcg – 500mcg is a standard starting dose.

See the Thyroid Protocol for more details.

B-Vitamins Biotin and Riboflavin

I'm putting these supplements near the end because they don't apply to everyone, but to certain individuals they are *extremely* important for clear skin.

If you struggle with "fungal" acne, dandruff, dermatitis, eczema, then biotin and riboflavin are crucial, *especially* if you are on a low-carb, ketogenic, or carnivore diet.

Both of these B-Vitamins are used in lipid transport, mobilization, and storage, and are crucial in making sure that your skin is healthy, moisturized, and able to combat natural threats.

Without adequate amounts of biotin and riboflavin, the skin

becomes cracked, dry, scaley, red, and suspectable to malassezia overgrowth that leads to fungal acne.

Because they are required for fat absorption, individuals consuming a high-fat diet (carnivore/ketogenic/low-carb) will require increased amounts of biotin.

If you are not consuming liver, salmon, or egg yolks on a regular basis, consider supplementing with 100mg of biotin and riboflavin. See The Fungal Acne Protocol for more information.

Probiotics

Bacteria play an essential role in our health, both inside the body and out.

The *gut microbiome*, or gut flora, is a massive colony of bacteria that influence a wide array of bodily functions, from digestion to stress control. Keeping this colony swimming with good, beneficial bacteria (probiotics) is crucial for clear skin.

- The gut flora protects the intestinal wall from leaky gut syndrome
- Probiotics break down many carbs and help with vitamin synthesis and absorption
- A healthy gut microbiome helps lower IGF-1, systematic inflammation, and oxidative stress which all cause acne

The problem with both oral probiotics and topical probiotics is that we still don't know what the ideal microbiome looks like. We have rough ideas, but with antibiotics, modern diets, and altered farming practices, it's impossible to know for sure. It's one of those really interesting "black boxes" within the medical community, and while we'll likely have a lot more knowledge of the ideal microbiome in the future, right now it's hard to pinpoint.

For this reason, the first step in creating a healthy gut microbiome should *always* be a healthy diet. If you're not giving probiotics the environment they need to thrive, you're going to be wasting your time and money. That's why before you start taking any probiotics, I recommend:

- Cutting out all grains and gluten
- Eating plenty of fresh vegetables, clean meats, and healthy fats
- Working on stress management wherever you can

If you want to have the added benefit of probiotics on top of that, here are a few that I recommend looking into. It's much better to be specific with your probiotics and target individual strains that help with acne, than take broad-spectrum probiotics that might actually throw your microbiome out of balance.

- Bacillus coagulan[68]
- Bifidobacterium bifidum[68]
- Bifidobacterium lactis[69]
- Enterococcus fecalis[70]
- Lactobacillus acidophilus[71]
- Lactobacillus bulgaricus
- Lactobacillus casei
- Lactobacillus paracasei
- Streptococcus salivarius[69]
- Bifidobacterium longum[72]

It may be hard to find these individual strains available for sale. Hyperbiotics® PRO-15 contains a large number of these strains, as well as a handful of other potentially anti-inflammatory probiotic strains as well. There is a new company called Skinesa® that also produces a highly-targeted probiotic for the skin. I am not affiliated with these companies in any way. I use Skinesa® daily, as it only contains a handful of useful strains in high quantities. Their early, double-blind clinical studies showed some pretty promising results when it comes to using probiotics for dietary-driven acne.

Again, probiotics are one of those things that are just a little too specific, a little too personal to be able to provide specific guidance on – the last thing I want to do is recommend a probiotic that actually makes your acne *worse*, which does happen. Skinesa® or Hyperbiotics® PRO-15 both seem to be pretty safe approaches, but do proceed with caution.

Other Harmless Supplements

The following supplements are likely to be non-impactful on acne but may be beneficial for your health. Don't sweat any of these supplements:

- Potassium
- Vitamin C
- Vitamin K
- Vitamin E (taken orally as it hasn't been shown to have a considerable impact on acne)

What About Other Supplements?

If you didn't see a supplement on the list above, I generally don't recommend taking it. Again, it's not that many of them are dangerous or harmful, just unnecessary. Most multivitamins, for instance, contain extremely high amounts of unnecessary vitamins that might actually make you less healthy and more prone to acne.

In my experience of helping hundreds of people along this journey, I highly recommend taking a "less is more" approach and focusing on getting nutrients through your diet whenever you can.

Chapter 12: Sleep, Stress, and Exercise

I said this at the beginning, but I'll repeat it here: this book is not going to contain an exercise program or meditation course. In this section, I'll give you a framework to help you think about these things, and what I believe are some of the most important lifestyle factors for clear skin.

What might work for one person might not work for another. Exercise is important, but how you get there isn't. If yoga is your thing, great. If weightlifting is your thing, awesome. Do what works for you.

Exercise

Exercise *can* play a very important role in helping with acne, but again, the main thing to remember here is that diet is key.

Look no further than bodybuilders with massive amounts of acne to see how more exercise does not necessarily mean less acne.

With that being said, exercise does touch all three of the root causes of acne:
- Decreases insulin resistance[73] (less hormonal acne)
- 20 minutes of moderate exercise leads to a decrease in inflammation throughout the body[74] (less inflammatory acne)
- It can positively impact the gut microbiome for better health[75] (less intolerance/digestive-driven acne)

Plus, exercise helps improve sleep quality, which we'll talk about shortly[76].

It's worth noting that the studies in question were using moderate exercise in twenty-minute spells – there's likely no need to push your body to the absolute limits to get these benefits. Just 15-20 minutes of solid movement a day can help a huge amount.

Weight training, cardio, yoga, breathwork, and even prolonged walking are all great ways to exercise – again, do what *you* enjoy.

There are research-based benefits to frequent movement[77], so while I'd recommend getting up and moving around at least once every 45 minutes to an hour, I'm also not going to advocate that you pick up an extreme exercise routine just to beat acne.

If that's your thing, then go for it - but again, even if you're exercising a ton, if your diet isn't in check then it won't matter. Exercise might give you a slightly larger buffer, per se, but it's not going to eliminate the negative side effects of a bad diet.

Stress Management

Stress is like inflammation – it's necessary for survival and (in small doses) can be a good thing.

For thousands of years, stress has triggered an inflammatory response that helps us fight off physical threats. This has been a necessary component of survival for all of human history.

But what about when that "threat" is traffic, social anxiety, or a work deadline? That's when you run into issues. Studies show that these minor psychological threats trigger pro-inflammatory responses that lead to chronic inflammation[78]. Stress also leads to the release of insulin and increased insulin resistance - yet another root cause of acne. Finally, stress negatively alters the gut microbiome[79].

What does this mean for you? Well, it means that chronic stress impacts all three root causes of acne – insulin, inflammation, and intolerance.

The key thing to remember is that *some* stress is good. *Some* stress is healthy. But it's only good when you *need* it, and most of us are triggering stress *far* too often.

The good news is that when you change your diet, adopt a simple exercise routine, and improve your sleep quality, your stress management skills will naturally start to improve.

Still, there are some things you can look into if you want to specifically target stress:

- Meditation
- Deep Breathing
- Reading
- Journaling
- Exercise
- Magnesium supplements
- Yoga

Source: Healthline

Sleep

Just like stress, sleep deprivation has a profound impact on your health, and touches all three root causes of acne:

- Sleep deprivation leads to increased inflammation and prevents our body from being able to properly trigger anti-inflammatory responses[80]
- Sleep deprivation leads to an increased insulin response[81]
- Sleep deprivation decreases the diversity and health of the gut microbiome[82]

The funny thing about sleep is that while our knowledge of it is growing, there still isn't a clear recommendation of how much sleep is necessary. If we're to trust the statistics, most of us are sleep deprived and in need of more sleep. Try to sleep as much as you can; the general consensus is at least 7 to 9 hours.

Some helpful tips that I've found useful include cutting down on screen time before bed, using blue light-blocking glasses as soon as the sun goes down, exercising, meditation, breathwork (inhale for 4 seconds, hold for 7 seconds, and exhale for 8 seconds), and supplementing with magnesium.

All of these factors are *interconnected*. They can work in either direction – stress, sleep, and exercise can either be a trigger for acne, or they can help you heal and prevent acne. It's hard to have success without all three.

Other Lifestyle Factors for Clear Skin

Here are a few loose ends that don't quite fit into the other categories. Some of these findings have research-backed evidence, while some of them are anecdotes that I've seen while working with people.

Ditch Your Fluoride Toothpaste

It's already bad enough that fluoride is a neurotoxin, but it also damages your thyroid and your skin. One study found that fluoride was responsible for "acne-like eruptions" on the skin[83], and several dentists claim that after having patients switch to non-fluoride toothpaste, their dermatitis, acne, and eczema subsided.

Furthermore, fluoride consumption over long periods of time (typically through tea or water, but also through our toothpaste, sublingually) is associated with a higher risk of thyroid disorders[84].

Meanwhile, rates of acne are sky-high for those with thyroid disorders. Basically, fluoride screws up your thyroid, and a screwed-up thyroid means acne.

Switch to a natural, fluoride-free alternative. I really like Jason Coconut Oil Mint, but there are tons of options out there that will work just as well.

Get *Some* Sun (and Ditch the Sunblock)

The sun is *amazing* tool to get clear skin. Not only does it replenish our body with vitamin D, which helps prevent inflammation, decrease insulin production, and improve digestion (all key factors for acne), it also can help act as a natural anti-bacterial and fungal defense on the skin.

We've been taught to be afraid of the sun and to lather up with tons of sunscreen, but it begs the question – what did our ancestors do for tens of thousands of years without sunblock?

One study found that over-exposure to sunlight affected less than one tenth of one percent of the global population negatively, while *under-exposure* to the sun (due to the fact most of us sit inside all day) affects *billions* of people, leading to autoimmune disorders (like acne)[85].

Definitely don't go out trying to get yourself burnt, but 20 minutes a day of unprotected sun exposure won't hurt. If you must use sunblock, go for a natural zinc oxide alternative, as many traditional sunblock brands are not only damaging to the skin's natural microbiome but also full of their own dangerous drawbacks. Burt's Bees make a natural face lotion with sunblock. Again, no sunblock or products is ideal, but it's a good solution if you know you'll be in a situation where you'd otherwise get burnt.

If you can't get 20 minutes a day of unprotected sun exposure, opt for a vitamin D3 supplement.

Filter your Water (if you can)

Remember how we were talking about fluoride earlier, and about how it impacts the thyroid and can cause acne?

Well, if you live in the United States, the odds are pretty good that your home tap water has fluoride in it. You can give it a Google; just search, "[MY CITY] fluoride water," and you should be able to find out.

While the amount of fluoride in tap water is relatively small, it can add up. In an *ideal* world, you could find a fluoride-free water source, but this isn't always possible. Reverse osmosis filters can run to several hundreds or even thousands of dollars, and buying spring water in bulk can get tiresome fast. This is one of those things that's great if you can afford it, but if not, don't sweat it – there are bigger battles to fight. Consider supplementing with iodine to counteract this, or purchase an alkaline water filter – they typically remove around 80% of the fluoride, which is better than nothing, and they're pretty cheap.

Chapter 13: Natural Skincare

This section is going to be short, mainly because it goes against the main philosophy of this entire book – clear skin from *within*.

Still, I understand that many people reading this book may feel uncomfortable with the idea of ditching their skincare routine cold turkey.

In the Root Causes section, we took a look at why the majority of acne products fail to work, and only really cover up the symptoms of acne. In this section, I'll outline a few strategies that you can use to bridge the gap from your current skincare routine to a natural skincare routine, or no skincare routine at all.

The Caveman Routine

In my opinion, it's honestly easiest to have an extremely minimal skincare routine and refrain from using any products.

There is a whole community of folks now who use nothing but water to wash their faces. My mother is one of them – she hasn't used soap or cleansers on her face for several years now.

This might sound unhygienic or gross, the but the truth is, for tens of thousands of years humans didn't have foamy cleansers, wipes, or miracle creams. We had water (often saline ocean water, which is anti-bacterial and anti-fungal) and sunlight.

Our skin, like our gut, has a natural microbiome of bacteria that protects it from outside threats. Using soaps, cleansers, and creams disrupts this gut microbiome and actually prevents healthy bacteria from being able to do their job. Sure, you might get rid of some acne bacteria, but in the long run you're only making it more challenging for your skin to survive on its own.

So, what exactly does a caveman routine look like?

- No soap, cleansers, creams, or products on the face
- Only water (saline water is acceptable and oftentimes helpful, cold water preferred)
- Minimal contact with shampoo or hair products

You can hypothetically wash your face with water as much as you'd like. I most commonly see people use a twice a day schedule, washing their face with water once at night and once during the day.

I know it sounds controversial, but I think you'd be surprised how beneficial this routine can be, and how amazing it feels to have such a simple routine. No more worrying about creams, cleansers, toners, etc. – it's very freeing.

Aloe Vera

So you still want to use some skincare products. I totally get that – from time to time, I'll use some as well, but I always make sure that they don't contain harmful agents that strip my skin of oils unnecessarily.

Aloe vera is a good example of a solid topical remedy with minimal negative side-effects.

Aloe vera is anti-inflammatory, kills bad bacteria, and promotes wound healing, which can heal acne scars at a much faster rate than if you didn't use aloe vera.

Ideally, the aloe vera you're buying should be natural, and this has very few potential downsides outside of allergies or irritation of the skin (which is why testing aloe vera on part of your face before slathering it all over is crucial).

Aloe vera isn't going to make up for an acne-causing diet, but it might help the healing process proceed a little bit quicker. The key is to make sure it's *real* aloe vera. When purchasing aloe vera, make sure that it's at least 99% aloe vera – there should be *very* few other ingredients. It should be liquid in composition, not extremely thick and gel-like. Use it once or twice a day for acne scars or faster healing.

Raw Honey

Raw honey is just awesome. It's anti-bacterial, anti-fungal, promotes wound healing, contains antioxidants that protect the skin, and acts as a moisturizer[86]. Honey first started being used for its topical medicinal purposes as a way to disinfect and promote wound healing in ancient civilizations, including Egypt.

It's dead simple, too – take some raw honey, stick a finger in, and create a thin layer across any area of the face, head, or chin that is prone to acne. Slathering honey on my face is one of the few topical treatments that I still use on occasion.

The key with using honey as a topical treatment is to use *raw*, *unpasteurized* honey. The anti-bacterial and anti-fungal benefits of honey come from the natural enzymes and compounds found in unheated honey. The pasteurization process kills these compounds and renders raw honey useless as a topical treatment (besides giving a moisturizing effect).

Pretty much any brand will do. I like to buy local. You'll probably here a lot of flak about how manuka honey is the best, but quite frankly I've found very little difference between extremely expensive manuka and my local bee farm's honey.

Salt Rinses

Alright, this one's a bit strange, but bear with me. Salt is one of the most powerful anti-fungal and anti-bacterial substances out there. I've read on numerous forums, discussion boards, and blogs about how simply swimming in the ocean once a day is a surefire way to cure dandruff and dermatitis. Unfortunately, most of us don't live near a salt-water swimming source, but we can simulate the effects of the ocean at home with some water and sea salt.

While acne is a bit different, it doesn't mean that the benefits of salt are totally void. Especially if you struggle with fungal acne, using salt can be an effective way to naturally destroy bad bacteria and fungi while maintain a healthy skin microbiome.

Simply mix a large portion of salt with water, and either spray, dab, rinse, wash, or submerge your face in or with the water. It's really that simple.

Apple Cider Vinegar

Apple cider vinegar is another tool that helps some people. Apple cider vinegar is also anti-bacterial and anti-fungal, and many people say that it helps them with fungal acne as well as regular acne. (I've used it for dandruff before, which is essentially the same thing.)

Take some apple cider vinegar and make sure you dilute it heavily with water – it shouldn't sting when you touch it. Apply gently to the face, and make sure you do a patch test with it (apply to one area of the face before proceeding with the whole face).

Again, this works for some people, and for others, not so much.

MCT Oil

MCT Oil *can be* a really powerful tool for beating not just regular, bacterial acne, but also fungal acne. While "fungal acne" actually isn't exactly "acne" (it's actually a form of atopic dermatitis caused by fungus as opposed to bacteria), many of the root causes remain the same. MCT oil, consisting primarily of capric and caprylic acid, is an extremely effective way to kill the Malassezia that triggers fungal acne.

The key is to make sure that the MCT oil you buy contains *only* capric acid and caprylic acid, and *not* lauric acid, because that actually can feed the fungus and contribute to worse acne.

Lather the face with a thin layer and wash off after 5-15 minutes.

Again, this is a little outside the scope of your typical acne infection, but may be a helpful tip for individuals dealing with dandruff or dermatitis alongside acne.

Topical Probiotics

Topical probiotics are extremely interesting, but just like oral probiotics, our knowledge of the skin microbiome is relatively limited (but growing fast). One company named Mother Dirt has created a probiotic spray that has shown to be effective at reducing acne over the course of a few months. One thing that's unclear is whether this change can be attributed to the probiotic spray itself or the fact that the individuals likely stopped using damaging acne products during this time. You can experiment with topical probiotics, but I wouldn't expect profound results from them.

What About "Fungal" Acne?

In the final section of this book, you'll find a full chapter on fungal acne and how it differs from regular, or "bacterial" acne, but since this is a dedicated space for topical treatments, I'll note some of the most common topical anti-fungal approaches.

In short, fungal acne is the byproduct of two things: overgrowth of the malassezia fungi on the skin, and an inflammatory reaction from the body in response to fungi itself. Whereas regular acne is the result of a bacterial infection and inflammation, fungal acne is the result of a fungal infection (or overgrowth) and inflammation.

Similarly, just like bacterial acne, our overall goal should be to stop fungal acne from within, addressing the inflammation head on using the dietary strategies outlined in the previous chapters. Fungal acne, however, is generally a bit harder to treat internally, and many people find that a single anti-fungal product can orient them in the right direction and speed up healing.

Sulfur

Sulfur powerful and relatively gentle anti-fungal substance that has been a huge aid for many individuals dealing with fungal acne.

You can get precipitated sulfur soap or sulfur ointment and use it once or twice a day. Look for 10% sulfur content and as few added ingredients as possible. Many people find soap in general to be drying, which further contributes to the red and irritated skin that accompanies fungal acne.

Zinc

Zinc is a great tactic to beat both bacterial and fungal acne internally, so it makes sense that it's also a great tool to beat it topically. You can use either zinc soap or cream.

In the case of zinc soap, look for something with few added ingredients and 2% pyrithione zinc. In the case of cream, look for "zinc oxide" (oftentimes sold as baby powder) with the fewest number of added ingredients.

Section V: Protocols

Protocols

Disclaimer: Information in this section is provided for informational purposes only. This information is not intended as a substitute for the advice provided by your physician or other healthcare professional. Do not use the information on this website for diagnosing or treating a health problem or disease, or with respect to starting, continuing, or ceasing any medication or other treatment.

This section is going to contain various specific protocols that you can use to get clear skin from within, no matter what your situation is. Each protocol will have a different overarching theme. Some of them will be based on dietary or ethical preferences, like the Vegetarian Protocol, while others will be based on your health or dietary goals, like the Thyroid Protocol.

Each protocol builds on what we've discussed in the previous sections and will contain not only where you should begin your elimination diet, but also which supplements you should consider.

While you don't necessarily have to follow any of these protocols, they can be helpful in narrowing down what works best for *you*.

Remember, the goal of these protocols is to get you on the right track so that you can find a diet and lifestyle that fits your needs, and your life – don't let these protocols take over your life or dictate your every move, they're just starting places.

Protocols Overview

There are quite a few chapters in this section, each aimed at a particular group of people who are struggling with unique acne-related issues. For this reason, I want to make sure that you can skip ahead to the protocol that you think best fits your particular situation:

- **Clear Skin Diet Blueprint** – Most people with mild to moderate acne should begin here. It's a good balance between being able to eat a wide variety of foods and overall health, and you can always jump to other protocols later if it's not working.
- **Insulin-Reduction Protocol** – If you struggle with severe acne *and* are consuming a medium to high amount of carbs in your current diet, you should consider this protocol.
- **Gut Protocol** – If you tried the Clear Skin Diet Blueprint and didn't experience the results you were looking for, this protocol can help you find those hidden triggers of acne.
- **Bacterial/Yeast Overgrowth Protocol** – If you've tried something like the Gut Protocol without results, it may be time to get tested for a fungal, bacterial, or yeast overgrowth, like candida or SIBO. Acne, dermatitis, and psoriasis are all common symptoms of these conditions.
- **Fungal Acne Protocol** – If you deal primarily with whiteheads, you may suffer from fungal acne, which requires a unique diet and topical approach.
- **Carnivore Protocol** – If you struggle with severe acne or have tried many other protocols without much success, the Carnivore Diet Protocol can be a very powerful tool, but is also hard to stick to.
- **Plant-Based Protocol** – Want to stick to a plant-based diet and still beat acne? No problem at all, we have a full section on it.
- **Thyroid Protocol** – Do you struggle with hormonal acne driven by your thyroid? This is particularly common for women. If so, this protocol will go over how to naturally treat thyroid-related acne for good.

Chapter 14: Clear Skin Diet Blueprint Protocol

The Clear Skin Diet Blueprint protocol takes everything we've covered so far in the book and puts it into a simple protocol so that you can get started in no time.

This protocol focuses on three key principles:

- Eliminating foods that trigger the root causes of acne for a period of time
- Eating anti-inflammatory and nutrient-dense foods that fight back against acne
- Listening to your body to figure out what works for you

The Clear Skin Diet Blueprint is called a "blueprint" for a reason – it's not something that's set in stone and which has to be followed *exactly*. Rather it should be used as a guide, or as a tool to start the journey towards clear skin. *Your* specific blueprint might actually look a lot different – you might find that you do better without macadamia nuts (a generally safe food) or that more carbs actually work *better* for your skin (most folks will want to be careful, but not *totally eliminate* carbs). This protocol is all about finding out what works for *you*.

Overview

The protocol has three main phases that we'll go through:

- Elimination phase (to find out what our main triggers of acne are)
- Testing phase (to find out what foods we can safely add back in)

- Optimization phase (to find out how we can make this diet work best for our lifestyle and preferences)

Expectations

One of the single most important things when going into a protocol like this is setting realistic expectations for yourself and the protocol as a whole.

If you are going to do the protocol, you need to commit for *at least two months.* The reason for this is simple: as we covered in the first section, the acne-forming process, from excess skin cell production to acne infection on the skin, takes about a month. You're going to want to give yourself another month to start really seeing dramatic results, and you might slip up along the way.

Still, with that being said, a lot of people notice markable improvements in as little as a week. Because inflammation is a huge factor in acne, creating swelling and redness, these visible symptoms can be diminished rather quickly.

I also want to note that things might get worse *before* they get better. While I've found this to be surprisingly uncommon, some folks actually add "healthy" foods that they haven't eaten in years and find that their body is intolerant to it. Others find the process itself stressful and get stress-related acne. That's why the key is to *commit to two months*, knowing that you *will* find what works for you during this time. If you see minor setbacks, don't stress - it's all part of the process and *you can do this*.

I know two months seems like a lot, but I can guarantee you that it'll be worth it in the long run. The body takes a long time to adjust, and if you give up after two or three weeks you might never really know whether or not you were on the right path. My own acne took about a month to show *any* signs of improvement, and then healed pretty rapidly. What would have happened if I had given up two weeks in? Well, I wouldn't be writing this book right now.

So, the key thing here is to stick with it and trust the process.

Phase I: Elimination

As I mentioned in the Diet section, a lot of folks worry about, "What should I eat, what superfoods should I add to beat acne?" This is the wrong approach to be taking. As we covered in the Root Causes section, our best bet at beating acne is to *eliminate* foods that are causing insulin, inflammation, and digestive-driven acne. That means that we're basically going to be sticking to the "Safe" foods from the Diet section, and *then* start incrementally adding back in foods that are safe but which may be common triggers of digestive issues or insulin production.

Because we broke down the foods in great detail in the Diet section, I'm not going to list *why* each food made the list. You can refer back to that section for that. Here I'm just going to outline a general recommended starting place for the elimination phase. This will be our "blueprint" for the first month.

Phase I: Safe to eat

- Meat (chicken and turkey in moderate amounts due to high inflammation-causing omega-6 content)
- Wild-caught seafood (if you can't get wild-caught, just don't eat seafood – farmed seafood is extremely high in inflammation-causing omega-6)
- Vegetables: pretty much all varieties, preferably lightly cooked in a healthy fat so the nutrients are more bioavailable and the antinutrients are diminished. See Diet section for more details.

- Fruit: pretty much all varieties, but again, see Section II for more details. You'll want to avoid having *too much* fruit, as some fruits are rather high in sugar, but they're all pretty easily digestible.
- Herbs and spices: rarely are there issues here.
- Healthy fats: coconut oil, MCT oil, ghee, olive oil, macadamia nut oil, tallow, etc.
- Safe starches in moderate amounts: white rice, sweet potatoes, squash, cassava, etc.
- Others:
    - Macadamia nuts
    - Coconuts
    - Olives
    - Avocados
    - Honey (in *small* amounts)

Basically, you're going to want to be eating *real foods* on this protocol. Think back to the diet we ate for the *vast majority* of human history in which we were hunter-gatherers – it was plants we could forage, and animals we could hunt. We didn't have wheat, soybeans, nutrition bars or fruit juices – we just had *real* foods that our body has evolved over tens of thousands of years to digest.

Phase I: Borderline foods

- Tea: tea is right on the edge, as it contains caffeine and can cause some issues, but is generally a lot safer than coffee because it's not as taxing on the digestive system and people are considerably less prone to intolerance issues
- Alcohol: if you can, remove alcohol from your diet, or at the very least, if you can't, opt for the healthier choices outlined in the Diet chapter
- Nightshades: potatoes that aren't sweet potatoes, tomatoes,

eggplants, goji berries, and peppers are all part of the "nightshade" family that are frequently said to cause autoimmune or inflammation issues – I would recommend cutting them out if you have *severe* acne and consume any of these foods regularly, but there's a lot of conflicting research

Phase I: Foods to Avoid

These are the foods you should *avoid* for Phase I. You *don't* have to give up these foods *forever*. Some of them, like gluten or sugar, you might *want* to, but please know going into this that the goal of Phase I is to determine which foods are causing your acne and what your triggers are. Once we understand this, we can start adding them back.

Is it going to be hard to give up these foods for a month? Yes. I won't lie to you and say that it's a breeze. Will it be worth it, and is it likely that along the way you'll find healthier alternatives that you enjoy, *and* that you'll both feel better and look better as a result? Yes.

So, bear with me here - we'll go over the order in which I recommend adding foods back in the next section.

- Grains: wheat, anything with gluten, barley, oats, cereal, quinoa, kernels, farrow, kasha, bulgur, pasta, bread, anything with "bran," etc.
- Corn: (corn syrup, especially high-fructose corn syrup, corn sweeteners, corn starch, corn oil, maize, etc.)
- Dairy besides ghee: again, don't sweat it if you just absolutely cannot live with dairy, but it's pretty important we cut it out for a while
- Beans and legumes of all varieties
- Nuts and seeds besides macadamias/coconuts: these are

extremely common intolerants – we'll be testing them out soon, as they're awesome sources of healthy monosaturated fats *if* you can tolerate them, but for now we need to stick to the safest of foods
- Any seed or vegetable oils (and any products containing these ingredients): corn oil, sunflower oil, canola oil, rice bran oil, sesame oil, peanut oil, cottonseed oil, sesame seed oil, safflower oil, margarine, shortening
- Coffee: I know, I know, but try switching to tea or caffeine capsules for the month! Seriously, coffee, even decaf, is sometimes the *single largest* factor in acne – it's such a widely used substance, yet an incredible amount of people are intolerant to it
- Anything with added sugar, which can appear in many forms
- Beverages: diet soda, fruit juice, alcohol - pretty much anything but water, coconut water, herbal tea, and if you have to, caffeinated tea
- Egg whites (extremely common intolerant, but if you *can* digest them well, the yolks are a great source of retinol vitamin A, vitamin D, vitamin E, and vitamin K)

Phew, so that's quite the list. If you want a really easy, straight-to-the-point PDF for this, go to https://goodglow.co/blueprint and download the blueprint. It's totally free and outlines everything that I've mentioned above in a single page.

Phase I: Macronutrients

We've talked about macros a lot, so I'll keep this short and sweet. If you want to really focus on cutting carbs to deal with hormonal acne, you can consult the Insulin Reduction Protocol or the Carnivore Protocol below.

In general, I don't think carbs are evil for most people, but we still need to make sure that we're avoiding *huge* insulin spikes. In this protocol, the foods most likely to do that are safe starches (white rice, sweet potatoes, etc.) and fruit, especially fruit that's high in sugar.

To avoid this, just don't go overboard on either. You don't have to count macros or anything like that (unless you want to), but maybe stick to a fistful or two of fruit at each meal, or a single serving of a safe starch per day.

Fat doesn't trigger a substantial insulin response (in fact it helps blunt it), so never worry about eating too much fat. Protein can actually trigger a minor insulin response, but again, it's not a worry for most people.

Key message here: don't overthink it.

Meal Timing

You probably know by now that I'm a huge proponent of focusing not just on *what* you eat, but also *when* you eat. Meal timing and frequency is an extremely important factor in all three root causes of acne: insulin production, inflammation, and digestive issues.

For this reason, I recommend you consider using this period to try out intermittent fasting (after talking to a healthcare professional, of course), if you haven't already – the easiest, most simple way is to start by skipping one meal. Eat two big, square meals throughout the day. Maybe it's breakfast at 7:00am and lunch at 2pm, or maybe it's lunch at noon and dinner at 6:00pm. Whatever you decide, try your best to eat two meals and *not snack* in-between meals. This gives your digestive system a much-needed break. If that's too challenging, you can try just having 3 meals a day with no snacking.

The reason I feel obligated to include this is that many people find that even after sticking to a rather strict diet, they are *still* getting acne. Then, all of a sudden, after picking up intermittent fasting things seem to improve, and improve rapidly.

You might have the perfect diet already, and instead of focusing on *what* you eat, you just need to focus on *when* you eat.

Phase I (and beyond): Supplements

I've covered supplements in greater detail elsewhere, so I'll just be brief here about what I think you should consider taking:

- **Vitamin A:** beef liver capsules if you're not eating liver
- **Vitamin D**3 if you're not getting 15 minutes of unprotected sun exposure a day
- **Zinc** if you're not eating a lot of lamb
- **Omega-3** (preferably algae-based or krill oil) if you're not eating wild-caught fish once or twice a week
- **Magnesium** (pretty much everyone should be taking magnesium)
- **Iodine** if you are continuing to drink tea
- **Biotin** and **riboflavin** if you are on a high-fat diet

Again, those are just the absolute essentials – you *can* take other supplements, but again, as I reference in the Supplements section, I don't think it's necessary or even beneficial in many cases.

Phase I: What about organic, or grass-fed, or pasture-raised?

Alright, so a lot of folks will draw attention to the whole "organic" vs. "conventional" debate, and "toxins," and how all these impact your body.

With the exception of factory-farmed fish versus wild-caught fish, I'm going to honestly say that I don't think it makes a substantial difference. It's infinitely better to eat a "non-organic" or "conventional" diet that's acne-friendly than it is to eat an organic acne-causing diet. There are dozens upon dozens of foods that are organic but awful for your skin.

If you can afford and find organic foods, pasture-raised meat, and wild-caught fish, then yes, totally go for it! Is it generally healthier? Yes (but in many cases it's negligible). Will it make or break your chances at clear skin? Absolutely not, and in a lot of cases it can actually hold folks back from starting to adopt the lifestyle changes they need to get clear skin.

Don't let the whole "organic" versus "conventional" game prevent you from making the changes that you want to see.

Phase I: Timeframe

Most trials conducted this sort of diet over a period of 6 weeks. You need to give your body time and space to adjust to the new diet, as you'll likely be going through some physiological changes as you adapt both physically and mentally to this diet.

I think that a really good benchmark for most people is 30 days. Set a goal, mark it on the calendar, and decide that for these 30 days you're going to take control of your health. 30 days is doable (there's a company called Whole30 that does 30-day diet challenges a lot like this), and it's an amount of time to follow something for which is enough for you to start seeing some real impact. Then, start Phase II of the process.

Phase II: Reintroduction

Alright, so you completed the month-long elimination phase, and hopefully your skin is already looking quite a bit better – if it's not, *that's okay*. We'll go over what to do if this is the case shortly.

Now, assuming that your skin is getting better, it's time to enter the re-introduction phase *if you would like to*. The reason I feel inclined to put this is that a lot of folks actually stick with this modified "Paleo" or "autoimmune-friendly" diet even after the initial 30 days. They feel so good that they want to stick with the plan they have in place. If that's the case (it was for me, but it certainly isn't for everyone) then you can use this section as a reference if you'd ever like to consider reintroducing foods.

For the rest of us who are eager to add back some foods and see how they affects our skin, there are two main things to consider here: which foods we should try reintroducing first, and how we should go about testing this.

Phase II: When to Reintroduce Foods

Reintroducing foods is a tricky subject, because some people will just choose not to, and that's *awesome*. But, if you want to reintroduce foods after the initial 30-day elimination, you might actually be better off waiting a bit more. Here are my general guidelines:

- If after the 30 days your acne is 90%+ eliminated and you want to reintroduce some foods, go for it!
- If your acne has improved significantly but still has a long way to go, consider sticking with the elimination protocol for another month and then reassess
- If your acne has not improved much or is still very severe, stick with the elimination protocol for as long as you can. If it continues to not improve, consider the Insulin

Protocol, Gut Protocol, or the Carnivore Protocol instead

There is no one-size-fits-all answer here, but one thing I *can* tell you is that, generally speaking, people *know* when it's the right time to start reintroduction. Again, a lot of folks don't even want to. That's just fine, too. Listen to your body and do what feels caring for yourself and your body.

Phase II: How to Reintroduce Foods

The basic protocol for reintroduction will go as follows:

- **Select:** Determine **one** food that you'd like to test, and commit to eating that food in *small* amounts two or three times in one day
- **Wait:** Do *not* eat that food again over the course of the next few days
- **Assess:** If you experienced a breakout, or your stomach hurt, or you had inflammation (joint pain, aching, etc.), then *do not proceed* with this food. You can try this food again later, as sometimes once the body has healed it becomes digestible again.
- **Eat:** If you did not experience any negative symptoms from your first day, eat another very small portion. Wait about a half hour. If you again experience no negative symptoms, eat a much larger, normal portion of the food.
- **Wait:** Wait about 5 days.
- **Assess:** If you experienced no symptoms, then you're good to try incorporating this back into your diet. If you did experience symptoms, wait another month and then you can try this food again if you still really want to eat it.

You should *not* be attempting to reintroduce multiple foods at once. I know the process seems painstakingly long, but it's really the only way to isolate the variables necessary to determine what's causing your acne – everyone's body is different, and this protocol will help *you* design a diet that works for *you*.

Here is a sample of what this might look like for reintroducing *almonds:*

- Monday: Eat two almonds
- Tuesday: Wait
- Wednesday: Wait
- Thursday: Did you experience a breakout? No? Then eat three or four almonds. Now, wait an hour or two. Still feeling good? Great. Now try having a handful or two of almonds. Nothing crazy, but a regular serving size.
- Friday: Wait
- Saturday: Wait
- Sunday: Wait
- Monday: Wait
- Tuesday: How'd the last few days go? Good? Great, try incorporating almonds back into your diet.

How do I know if I'm intolerant to a certain food?

A lot of folks ask, "How can I know if a certain food is hard for me to digest?" There are a lot of signs, and at the end of the day you're the only one who can know for sure, but I always like to remind people that digestion also relies on our body's autonomic nervous system - in other words, whether we're in fight-or-flight (sympathetic) or rest-and-digest (parasympathetic) mode. If you're eating a new food and thinking, "Oh my god, this is going to kill me!" before you even take the first bite, then you might be psyching yourself out.

I'm not trying to imply that food intolerances are as simple as shifting your mindset – they're not - but try to go into each reintroduction as calmly as possible and be willing to accept your body's response in either *direction* – on the other end of the spectrum, I see a lot of folks trying to justify foods or drinks (especially coffee) that make them feel and look terrible.

Here are a few common symptoms:

- Breakouts – surprise, surprise, acne, pimples, etc. are an easy way to determine your tolerance to a particular food, but this *only works* if you were previously on an elimination diet and reintroduced a single food – otherwise, breakouts could be due to any number of factors
- Eczema, dandruff, or psoriasis
- Abnormal joint pain or muscle discomfort
- Stomach aches or pain
- Diarrhea, extremely loose stools, or large amounts of undigested food in the stool
- Fatigue (more than the usual afternoon slump)
- Brain fog (again, most of us get brain fog from time to time, so we're talking about an acute instance after eating the food)

Again, listening to your body and being honest about your reaction is key here.

Phase II: Which Foods to Reintroduce

When reintroducing foods, it's important to ask yourself a few questions: first, why are you reintroducing a certain food? Is it because you love the taste of that food? Is it because some blogger told you it's the new superfood? Is it because your gut tells you that you should be eating it? Thera are a lot of reasons to attempt reintroduction, and understanding why you want to reintroduce a food is just as important as the process that goes behind it.

If you want to reintroduce cereal because the sugar rush gets you going in the morning, maybe it's time to reconsider your choice and see if you could replace that cereal with some fruit. Alternatively, if your body is screaming, "Get me some almonds!" then it might be time to listen to it.

Introducing safer foods is always ideal, but at the same time, the Elimination Phase can be quite strict. Whenever possible, go for Safe-to-Moderate foods (again, you can download a one-page summary on goodglow.co/blueprint) for reintroduction, and if you're attempting to add in unsafe foods, then try your best to find moderate alternatives that fit the bill. Dark chocolate (80%+ cacao), for instance, isn't a great choice for many people, but it's a *much* better choice than a candy bar.

Here are some of the safer foods to attempt reintroducing:

- Moderate amounts of nuts and seeds (*not* peanuts/peanut butter, which are legumes)
- Nightshades (potatoes [besides sweet potatoes, which were already allowed], peppers, goji berries, etc.)
- Higher-FODMAP foods (if you previously cut them out)
- Egg whites (awesome if you can tolerate them, pasture-raised is ideal, this makes a big difference in eggs)
- Coffee
- Dark chocolate (high-cacao - a simple hack is to look for stevia-sweetened dark chocolate to blunt the insulin spike)
- *Some* raw, full-fat, preferably grass-fed dairy (sheep/goat cheese, butter, kefir, and cream)
- Potatoes (besides sweet potatoes, which are fine even during the elimination period)

While many foods are relatively safe to reintroduce, there are a lot of foods that I'd recommend that you try and find alternatives to, simply by virtue of the fact that they trigger more than one of the root causes of acne, and quite profoundly:

- *Most* dairy (all milk, low-fat or non-raw yogurt, cheese, ice cream)
- *Most* grains/starches (soy, wheat, corn, oats, buckwheat, quinoa)
- Fruit juice (just pure sugar), soda (including diet)
- Anything with added sugar
- Any vegetable or seed oils (see Blueprint for full list)
- Beans and legumes, especially if not soaked and properly prepared

Basically, if it's not a whole food that you could find in nature without needing to process (e.g. grains/beans), consider trying to find an alternative.

Phase III: Maintenance & Optimization

Phase III can come as early as a month after starting or take as long as six months. If you find that the Elimination Phase diet works for you, then you might arrive here pretty quickly. If you've really had a hard time reintroducing food, or started the process with severe acne, it could take a bit longer to get here.

There are two paths for Phase III:

- **Maintenance** – find better, easier ways to stick to what you've built so far
- **Optimization** – tweak, refine, and alter your program for better results

Some folks coming into Phase III are going to be ecstatic and happy with the diet and lifestyle that they've built for themselves, and furthermore, with their skin. At this point, you should have had markable improvements in your complexion (on a 10-point scale, an improvement of 7 or 8). If this is you, then your path is **maintenance** – we want to do everything we can to make sure you that you keep on making solid progress and building on the habits you've started.

If you are unhappy with your results and are eager, wiling, and ready to take the next step, then **optimization** is the path for you. Here, I want to make something clear - **optimization** for *most* people isn't necessary, but there are some folks who need to adopt an even stricter elimination diet or deal with specific health issues (thyroid-driven acne, for instance). Choose which path you think fits where you're at, and you can always return here later.

Phase III: Maintenance

The goal of a maintenance strategy is to make sure that you can keep living the lifestyle that you've built for yourself over the following months, years, or *even* decades.

Now, while I'm not a psychologist or behavioral expert, I am someone who has helped a lot of different people take control of their skin from within, and I've started to learn from experience what works and what doesn't work.

Surprisingly, what *doesn't* work is willpower, motivation, and discipline. If you have to whip yourself into shape each and every time you eat vegetables or mentally chastise yourself every time you see a doughnut, this isn't going to work long-term for you.

On the contrary, doing the elimination diet in Phase I for a month *is* possible through determination and willpower. You can just power through those 30 days. But, unless you enjoy and *want* to continue with your clear skin lifestyle, it simply won't work over a longer term. That's why you need to find foods, activities, and techniques that fit your own goals and desires.

This could be as simple as having a cup of green tea (assuming you reintroduced it successfully) in the morning instead of telling yourself you'll only drink water. Or, instead of allowing your anger and resentment build up to an ultimate cheat meal of a giant pizza, allowing yourself to have some raw goat cheese instead. Again, I can't tell you what strategies specifically will work, as the "borderline" foods that you can tolerate will be different, but it's much better to "cheat" with a food that you can tolerate and which satisfies your craving than it is to get so frustrated that you can't adhere to your own rules.

If you are forcing yourself to do this, it's time to start looking for little ways that won't impact your skin to help you along this journey. This protocol is an outline, a guide for what *might* work for you, not a code that you *need* to follow.

I know this has been rather vague, but I truly think that this is perhaps the most important lesson in the book – *you* need to *want* to follow your own dietary and lifestyle choices, otherwise it's simply not going to work.

Phase III: Optimization

Alright, so you're either not quite happy with your results, or you feel so good that maybe you want to push your performance and wellbeing even further. You're in the right place.

There are a few reasons that you might not be achieving the results you want, and I've laid out protocols for each of them. If you're happy with what you've got, then great, but if not, here is where I'd recommend starting:

- **Insulin-Reduction Protocol:** If during your Elimination Phase you were *still* eating a generous amount of carbs, consider this protocol
- **Gut Protocol:** If you seem to be sensitive to even the foods on the Elimination list, this may be a good place to

start which isn't as extreme as the Carnivore Protocol
- **Carnivore Protocol:** A rather intense and extreme protocol, but also a powerful one for severe acne and other autoimmune conditions
- **Fungal Acne Protocol:** If you're dealing primarily with pus-filled white heads and dry, itchy, flakey skin (especially on a keto/carnivore diet), you may have fungal acne
- **Thyroid Protocol:** This is unique and specific to thyroid issues - consider looking into it if you frequently feel cold, lack energy, and struggle with jawline acne
- **Plant-Based Protocol**: If you want to remain plant-based while beating acne, this is the place to go

In addition to these protocols, I'll refer you to two sections:

- **Fasting section** – consider implementing intermittent or prolonged fasting to really supercharge your results
- **Lifestyle and supplements** – diet and fasting gets us 90% of the way there, but supplements and your lifestyle can help too

Chapter 15: Insulin Reduction Protocol

The Insulin Reduction Protocol is a framework for a few different types of folks:

- You tend to break out after eating sugary foods, or even rich carbohydrates like sweet potatoes, white rice, yam, etc.
- You are prediabetic or want to lose weight while beating acne
- You feel better eating fewer carbs, or you're intrigued by the benefits of a low-carb or ketogenic diet

I generally recommend that people start with the Clear Skin Diet Blueprint, but there's no harm in utilizing this program if you really want an added boost.

The goal of this program is simple: eat a diet and live a lifestyle that promote a healthy insulin response.

You'll remember that insulin is the hormone that gets triggered after we eat food – it helps convert sugar in the bloodstream into usable energy for the body. It's a necessary component of our hormonal health. Unfortunately, *too* much insulin, which can be triggered by eating certain foods (primarily foods high in carbohydrates) can cause a cascading effect of biological reactions which cause acne:

- Excess production of sebum oil, which can clog pores
- Increased inflammation, which contributes to pimples and acne
- Increased production of skin cells, which will eventually

rise to the surface of the skin and block pores

Upwards of *half* of Americans have insulin resistance, which means they produce a huge amount of this acne-causing hormone[87]. It's no wonder that rates of acne are also at all-time highs across the United States.

I won't go into all the science again - you can refer to the first section for the full details - but the goal of this diet is to *limit* the consumption of foods that trigger significant insulin spikes. To do this, we'll adopt a low-carb, or "ketogenic" diet. Basically, instead of relying on carbohydrates from our food for energy, we'll metabolize our own body fat (and dietary fat, too) as energy and avoid the huge ups and downs of insulin spikes.

Now, I know that sounds awfully scary, and there are a lot of conflicting viewpoints about keto out there, but I really want to assure you that low-carb diets are one of the best ways to reduce acne. In fact, low-carb diets are amongst the only research-based diets we have that are proven to *significantly* improve acne.

One comprehensive study on the effects of the ketogenic diet found that insulin resistance dropped by upwards of 75% after *just two weeks* of eating a low-carb diet[88].

Keto not only reduces insulin spikes which trigger hormonal acne, but it also reduces inflammation[89]. Add in some gut-friendly and easily digestible foods, and you have yourself a diet that combats all three root causes of acne. It really is one of the most powerful and useful diets out there for fighting acne.

FAQ: Isn't low-carb or keto just eating fats and oils? Can I not eat out at restaurants anymore?

If you're extremely turned off the idea of keto, I get it – a lot of folks think that you have to eat sticks of butter and mounds of ground beef just to get by, and never eat a plant again. I'm here to assure you, as someone who did keto for over two years, that this is *not* the case. You *can* survive off coconut oil and fatty meat, but you can also follow this protocol and enjoy delicious meals with nuts, seeds, meat, seafood, vegetables of just about every variety, some fruit, and even dark chocolate.

Again, I recommend coming to this protocol *after* the Clear Skin Diet Blueprint Elimination Phase so that you know which foods you can tolerate, but I just want to assure you that the Insulin Reduction Protocol is anything but boring and it's becoming easier and easier to do at restaurants and while traveling. It takes some getting used to, but honestly I found keto considerably easier than people make it out to be, and I'll break down why in this section.

What to eat: Macronutrients

Our goal with this diet is to avoid foods that trigger significant insulin spikes so that we can avoid hormonal acne. For the most part, that means we'll be sticking to foods that are higher in fat, moderate or low in protein, and low in carbohydrates.

Unlike the Clear Skin Diet Blueprint, where the focus was more on what you ate but not necessarily the specific macronutrients, the Insulin Reduction Protocol does require that you are aware of your "macros": carbs, fat, and protein.

For the most beneficial effects, you're going to want your body to be in "ketosis" or a fat-burning state. The reason for this is that being in ketosis can reverse insulin resistance and lead to that anti-inflammatory effect we discussed earlier. To do this, you'll need to eat **fewer than 20g of net carbs per day.** Net carbs are simply "Total Carbohydrates" minus "Dietary Fiber," as fiber is technically a carbohydrate but doesn't trigger an insulin response from the body (the body can't use fiber as energy, or really even digest it, for that matter).

So, if a protein bar has a whopping 17g of carbohydrates, but 15g are in dietary fiber, then it would really only be 2g of "net carbs," and you could safely have 18g of other net carbs throughout the day. It's worth noting that everyone will get "kicked out" of ketosis by different things, so 20g is just a generally recommended baseline, not a set-in-stone rule.

Furthermore, there is still a *huge* amount of benefit to eating a small but non-ketogenic amount of carbs. We can break down the Insulin Reduction Protocol into two categories:

- **Ketogenic:** Fewer than 20g of net carbs per day (or 5% of total calories)
- **Low-Carb:** Fewer than 50g of net carbs per day

Both are going to have huge benefits for your skin. While I'd recommend the ketogenic diet for individuals struggling with intense acne, if you have a hard time doing fewer than 20g then you can still reap many of the benefits at fewer than 50g.

Furthermore, on a true ketogenic diet, you should try to keep your protein to around 25% of your total calories. The reason for this is that while fat doesn't trigger an insulin response from the body, protein still does, just not to the same degree that carbohydrates do. What that means is that *most* of your calories should be coming from high-fat foods, *if* you want to stay in ketosis. Too much protein will actually throw you out of ketosis.

Again, it's totally up to you, but that's the general guideline for achieving the medically proven benefits of ketosis.

FAQ: How do I know how many net carbs I've eaten?

The first step is to start looking at nutrition labels (or Google for foods nutrition values). Take total carbs, subtract fiber, and you've got **net carbs**. You'll start to get a feel for how many carbs foods typically have.

You do *not* have to track your macros down to the smallest degree forever. In fact, I find that to be a huge turnoff for a lot of people starting keto. Instead, what I recommend doing is downloading an app like Chronometer and tracking what you eat (and drink) for *three* or *four* days after you get into the habit of eating low-carb and know what your typical day looks like. You'll pretty quickly get an idea for where you're at and be able to make any adjustments to get you in the zone you want. If you found tracking your macros to be helpful, you can continue doing it, but most people find it unnecessary.

FAQ: How do I know if I'm in ketosis?

Don't worry about it. Honestly. I know that sounds like bad advice, but it's a rabbit hole that is honestly not worth going down. You can buy urine strips and prick your finger with blood ketone monitors, but for most people it's just not worth it. Are you sticking to fewer than 20g of net carbs per day, *without* cheat meals? Then you'll be in ketosis once your body becomes fat adapted (this can happen within a matter of days, or take months – just stick with it).

If you enjoy knowing whether or not you're in ketosis, or what your blood ketone levels are, then by all means go for it. I just have found that for the majority of people I work with, tracking macros after the first few weeks and monitoring ketone levels are just not worth it and make the process discouraging and hard.

What to eat: Foods

Generally speaking, a typical ketogenic or low-carb diet will consist of the following low-carb foods:

- Meat (fattier is ideal) – beef, lamb, pork, poultry, turkey, etc.
- Fish & seafood (fattier is ideal) – salmon, sardines, trout, shrimp, shellfish, oysters
- Eggs
- Whole-fat dairy
- Leafy vegetables – spinach, romaine, broccoli, kale, cauliflower
- Healthy fats – coconut oil, butter, olive oil
- Nuts – almonds, macadamias, pecans
- Zero-calorie beverages (besides diet soda, which triggers insulin) – water, coffee, tea, etc.

While this is a pretty good start, some of these foods, like whole-fat dairy, vegetable oils, or even nuts, can cause a lot of problems for people with acne.

The key for the perfect Insulin Reduction diet is to combine low-carb foods with anti-inflammatory *and* easily digestible foods. Basically, what we're going to do is take the Clear Skin Diet Blueprint and select only the low-carb options. In order to do this, we need to remove a few foods that are "technically" allowed on your average ketogenic diet…

1. Avoid vegetable oils (canola, corn, soybean, sunflower, safflower, etc.) and stick to the following healthy fats: olive oil, coconut oil, avocado oil, beef tallow, and grass-fed ghee. Vegetable and seed oils are loaded with omega-6 fatty acids which can trigger inflammatory acne.
2. Avoid all dairy except for grass-fed ghee and grass-fed butter if you can tolerate it. All other forms of dairy, despite seeming to be low in carbs, actually trigger a huge insulin spike due to the lactose found in dairy. In fact, milk

can trigger a more significant insulin spike than many other carb-heavy foods.
3. Don't eat too many nuts as many of them are high in omega-6 fatty acids. Treat them like a snack, and stick to nuts low in omega-6 like macadamias, hazelnuts, or almonds.
4. Test whether or not you can eat eggs. Egg yolks are an amazing form of nutrition, but many people are intolerant or allergic to egg whites.
5. Avoid processed foods whenever possible. Even many "healthy" keto bars or snacks are loaded with inflammation-causing omega-6 fatty acids. When in doubt, refer to the Clear Skin Diet Blueprint.

Again, using the Clear Skin Diet Blueprint in conjunction with this protocol is ideal as you'll avoid inflammatory and gut-damaging foods, and it will provide a good starting place for the most common mistakes to avoid.

Intermittent Fasting

This is going to be the only protocol where intermittent fasting is an explicitly mentioned aspect of the protocol. When it comes improving your body's insulin response, intermittent fasting is one of the most beneficial tools out there. If you consult with a healthcare professional and it's determined that intermittent fasting is safe for you, then consider starting with the 16/8 intermittent fasting (skip breakfast) or the 5:2 (eat normally 5 days a week and fast for 2). Refer to the Fasting chapter for more details, but just know that this diet in particular is fasting-friendly as you'll be avoiding the constant blood sugar spikes that make you hungry.

Supplements

I recommend the same supplement strategy here as the Clear

Skin Diet Blueprint, but I want to emphasize the importance of electrolytes on any low-carb diet. Your body will deplete electrolytes rapidly, so supplement with the following:

- Potassium – supplements (or use "Lite Salt")
- Sodium – just adequately salt your food and have a tiny bit of salt in the morning, even if you're fasting
- Magnesium – use magnesium chloride or another magnesium supplement

Additionally, getting enough biotin and riboflavin is absolutely essential on a ketogenic diet, and without them, you make yourself suspectable to fungal acne, dermatitis, and dandruff.

Both biotin and riboflavin are nutrients that are involved in fat transport. They help your body store and use fat for energy. The more fat you consume, the more biotin and riboflavin your body requires. Because ketogenic diets are naturally high in fats, this means the requirement for biotin increases.

Without biotin and riboflavin, the skin cannot receive the lipids it needs to be properly protected and healthy, leading to cracked, red, dry, flakey skin. This is the perfect breeding ground for fungi and yeast overgrowth that can lead to fungal acne.

Unfortunately, there aren't too many low-carb foods that are high in biotin and riboflavin except egg yolks (avoid the whites, they bind to biotin and make your body unable to absorb it), salmon, and organ meats. For this reason, if you are not eating egg yolks, salmon, or organ meats once a week, you will want to consider adding 100mg of biotin and riboflavin per day.

See the Fungal Acne Protocol for more information.

FAQ: How long should I stick with it?

I alluded to this earlier - there is a process in which your body will transition from burning primarily carbs for fuel to burning primarily fat for fuel. **This process takes time.** You might not feel so great and your skin might not look amazing for the first few weeks. If you're experienced with fasting or you've dabbled in low carb diets before, then this process might happen quite rapidly. The aforementioned study demonstrating the benefits of a low-GI diet for acne showed significant improvements in just a few weeks.

Still, if you've been eating a lot of carbs for a very long time, the transition period might take a while. That's totally normal. Keep sticking with it, and give yourself at least two months before you ditch the protocol.

FAQ: Can I have cheat meals?

Let's say you want some carbs. What will happen?

Well, you'll be kicked out of ketosis, you'll likely feel pretty lethargic, and your body will trigger a significant insulin spike.

Will it kill you? Absolutely not. Will it cause acne? Maybe; this really depends on how long you've been doing a low-carb diet, how you react to carbs, what your cheat meal was, etc.

Whenever possible, eat a cheat meal of carbs with *healthy*, anti-inflammatory and gut-friendly foods: fruits, sweet potatoes, cassava, etc.

There is something called a cyclical ketogenic diet, where individuals eat a high-carb meal once or twice per week, but for the vast majority of people a standard, sustainable low-carb diet is ideal. Trust me - when you cheat, it's harder to get back on the bandwagon. These modified approaches are generally recommended for athletes.

FAQ: What about alcohol?

Most alcohol is high in carbs or sugar, meaning it's not low-carb friendly. Still, there are dry wines, hard liquor (with nothing else added), and other low-carb alcohol alternatives that are relatively keto-friendly. Great choices for your skin? Probably not, but you don't have to just give up alcohol - there are definitely better choices. See the diet section for more info.

Chapter 16: Gut Protocol

The Gut Protocol is for individuals who have tried the Clear Skin Diet Blueprint or a similar autoimmune/Paleo diet and *still* struggle with acne. Specifically, the gut protocol is for individuals who also experience autoimmune symptoms like dandruff, eczema, dermatitis, psoriasis, itching, rashes, indigestion, or irritation, especially after meals. What this protocol is going to aim to do is eliminate all but the most easily digestible foods, and then add back foods incrementally to find the triggers. The protocol is ideal for:

- If you've used antibiotics a lot in the past
- If you have tried rather extreme or strict diets and experienced improvements in your skin, but still can't shake the acne

Please note, if you *think* you are struggling with Candida, small intestinal bacterial overgrowth (SIBO), small intestinal fungal overgrowth (SIFO), or other yeast, bacteria, or fungal-related overgrowth, I actually recommend trying this protocol first to see if you can alleviate the issue. These disorders are difficult to pin down, and even natural remedies to combat these issues can do more harm than good. For this reason, I always recommend trying to avoid taking any form of antibiotics (including "natural" forms, like oregano oil) and fixing the issue with a diet-first approach. The good news is that this protocol will eliminate the primary dietary drivers of Candida, SIBO, and SIFO.

If you have tested positive for Candida, SIBO, or SIFO, have tried the Gut Protocol or Clear Skin Diet Blueprint, *and* are looking for an alternative to prescription antibiotics (great choice!), then refer to the Fungal Acne & Bacterial/Yeast Overgrowth Protocol. I always recommend that people proceed with caution here.

Protocol Overview

This is going to be a more targeted version of the Clear Skin Diet Blueprint, so that we can *really* pin down what might be causing these digestive issues. This protocol will look similar:

- Phase I: Elimination
- Phase II: Reintroduction
- Phase III: Maintenance & Optimization

Phase I: Elimination

While the Clear Skin Diet Blueprint is a great starting place for many people, if you're *still* struggling after several months, it means there's likely an underlying issue that's causing gut problems. This can be as simple as a single food that causes an inflammatory response, or as complex as something like candida or SIBO. The good news is that the Clear Skin Diet Blueprint is already a solid starting place for both of these types of issues, and we just have to make a few modifications.

In addition to all the recommended foods to cut out on the Clear Skin Diet Blueprint, cut out the following foods for 30 days:

High FODMAP foods

FODMAPs are fermentable carbohydrates that *certain people* have a hard time digesting. The bacteria in these carbohydrates can cause indigestion and IBS. FODMAPs themselves don't trigger an *immune* response, which means they won't directly cause an autoimmune response that leads to acne, but they *can* contribute and exacerbate other digestive issues, like SIBO, which can contribute to acne, dermatitis, or eczema. For this reason we'll eliminate them temporarily, but add them back when we get back control of our microbiome.

High-FODMAP foods include:

- Vegetables: Asparagus, artichokes, onions, leeks, garlic, beans, lentils, chickpeas, sugar snap peas, beets, cabbage, celery, corn, avocado, cauliflower, mushrooms, Brussels sprouts, fennel, okra, peas, shallot, radicchio
- Fruits: Apples, pears, mango, watermelon, nectarines, peaches, plums, cherries,
- Grains: Rye, wheat, semolina, couscous, bulgur
- Nuts: Cashews, pistachios
- Condiments: Honey, agave, relish, jam, tahini, tzatziki dip, hummus

Tea, Coffee, Mate

Tea and coffee are common intolerants. Coffee more so than tea, but it's important that you cut them both out for just this period. I know, this is tough, but this protocol is meant for folks who have struggled with acne for quite some time now, and for a lot of people coffee or tea is the last building block to get rid of acne. No caffeine is ideal, but if you must, go with a caffeine capsule and swap tea or coffee with a herbal tea or herbal coffee alternative.

Alcohol

Alcohol has to be cut out at this stage. It's linked with higher rates of eczema and psoriasis, and if you want to *truly* test this protocol out, you need to figure out if alcohol is triggering your acne. If you aren't able or don't want to do this, that's just fine, but then I recommend adjusting your expectations for the protocol accordingly.

Nightshades

Potatoes that aren't sweet potatoes, tomatoes, eggplants, goji berries, and peppers

Limit Safe Starches

Even though sweet potatoes, white rice, cassava, and the other safe starches are low-FODMAP, there's speculation that the relatively high carb content may still contribute to Candida. I don't think it's necessary to completely cut out sweet potatoes or yam, but don't go overboard on them either.

High-Histamine Foods

High-histamine foods may be the cause of your digestive issues or contribute to underlying gut issues, especially in the case of bacterial or fungal issues. Again, we need to cut these foods out just long enough to determine which of these groups is causing our underlying issues:

- Alcohol
- Fermented foods (kimchi, sauerkraut, kombucha, etc.)
- Dried fruits
- Avocados which are more than a day past peak ripeness
- Eggplant
- Spinach
- Processed or smoked meats
- Shellfish

Limit High-Oxalate Foods

Again, as we covered in the Diet section, oxalates *typically* aren't an issue, and individuals will be fine adding them back in, but for the time being you should avoid eating *raw* kale, spinach, chard, or other leafy green vegetables. It's fine to consume these in moderate amounts after light cooking, but I still wouldn't recommend going overboard.

Summary

Alright, so I know this leaves you with a rather limited list, but bear in mind that the goal here is to determine which main group is causing your digestive issues so that you can reintroduce the other groups. Here is a general list of "safe" foods for this initial period:

- Meat – preferably cooked immediately upon thawing to avoid histamine
- Wild-caught seafood
- Organ meats (amazing for their micronutrient content)
- Macadamia nuts
- Olives
- Coconut
- Avocados (fresh, not too far past ripeness)
- Healthy fats: Olive oil, coconut oil, beef tallow, avocado oil, ghee (avoid butter for this phase)
- Low-FODMAP vegetables (see above for full list to avoid)
- Small to moderate amounts of LOW-FODMAP, low-sugar fruits (see above for full list to avoid)
- Small amounts of safe starches (sweet potatoes, white rice, cassava, yam, pumpkin, etc.)
- Beverages: water, herbal tea, sparkling water

Stick to this for 30 days before moving on to Phase I – it's crucial that we can determine what the underlying cause is *before* we start adding back each problematic group.

Phase II: Reintroduction

Alright, so now that the 30 days are complete, you have hopefully experienced a pretty intense change in your skin. This is a rather extreme protocol, so if you *haven't*, then it might be time to start looking into some alternatives – adding more organ meats, going low-carb, carnivore, implementing intermittent fasting, etc.

Still, I want to stress that this should *not* be a psychologically stressful process. You should never feel like the diet itself is causing more stress than just eating other foods was. Your body and mind are intimately connected, and stress actually greatly hampers your ability to digest certain foods.

While I never recommend "cheating" or "quitting," I also don't recommend adopting a diet that makes you miserable, stressed out, or constantly paranoid that certain foods will make you break out. I truly hope that isn't the case, and if it is, then don't worry, because during this reintroduction phase we're going to start adding back foods pretty quickly.

We're going to follow the same one-week reintroduction protocol to that of the Clear Skin Diet Blueprint – so, basically, we'll take a week or so to reintroduce some foods, but this time we're going to do it a bit more tactically.

Try reintroducing foods in the following order, based on the list of foods to avoid above:

- Week 1: A high-FODMAP food (if you can tolerate FODMAPs, you'll open yourself up to *way* more dietary options)
- Week 2: A high-histamine food
- Week 3: A nightshade
- Week 4: Coffee/Tea/Mate

You're free to do this in whatever order, but I generally recommend this order because you start with foods least likely to cause issues (most people are fine with FODMAPs) and go towards foods that a larger proportion of the population have a hard time with (coffee/tea/mate).

It's key that for each week, you choose a *single food* from that group that you'd like to add back in, and follow the structure outlined in Phase II of the Clear Skin Diet Blueprint.

While it sounds counter-intuitive, the goal here is actually to figure out which group is causing you issues and to do so quickly. If you identify that high-histamine foods are what was triggering your symptoms, then you have your new, personalized Diet Blueprint and you're good to go (after following this reintroduction process for the other foods).

Phase III: Maintenance and Optimization

Okay, so now we're in familiar territory – did the protocol work? Did you find what was triggering your digestive issues?

If so, then I'm hoping this has provided you with your own little framework to follow, and also a method that you can come back to at any time.

If it *didn't,* then it's time to consider a few things.

First: how are you doing mentally and physically? I know this sounds silly, but if this process is causing you to become extremely stressed out, I *don't* think you should keep diving into more and more extreme protocols. You can always try something like the Carnivore Diet, but it if you're extremely stressed out by this whole ordeal, you honestly might just need a mental reset, or to try going back to something like the Clear Skin Diet Blueprint and giving it more time.

On the contrary, if your spirits are high and you maybe experienced *some* results, but not the exact results you were hoping for, I would point you in a few directions:

1. Combine this with the Insulin-Reduction Protocol (low-carb)

2. Check out the Carnivore Protocol
3. Check out the Thyroid Protocol (if you can get your thyroid tested, you may be dealing with hormonal acne that changing your diet can help but not necessarily cure)
4. If your acne is primarily pus-filled white heads or you also struggle with dandruff, check out the Fungal Acne Protocol
5. Refer to the Fasting chapter

Again, these are just points of reference. It may make sense to see a naturopath or dietician, too. This is rarely the case after adopting a protocol like this, but some people may be dealing with an underlying issue that can't be addressed through diet alone.

Chapter 17: Bacterial/Yeast Overgrowth Protocol

In addition to your run-of-mill food intolerances that can cause acne, there are also certain digestive issues, usually a result of bacterial, fungal, or yeast overgrowth that can cause not just acne, but also dermatitis, psoriasis, and eczema.

Some of these include Candida, small intestinal bacterial overgrowth (SIBO) and small intestinal fungal overgrowth (SIFO), among others. The most common approach to treating these issues is with diet and natural antibiotic and antifungal medications.

Before we dive into this protocol, we need to go over a very necessary and extremely important disclaimer.

There are a lot of instances in which antifungals, antibiotics, and probiotics are necessary to improve gut health. If you've taken antibiotics quite frequently in the past, or even as a child, this may be a necessary addition to the protocol.

Still, if you're struggling with gut issues, I'd recommend adding high-quality probiotics *alongside* a strong diet. Just like everything in life, more isn't necessarily better when it comes to probiotics – many of the leading probiotics actually contain small amounts of the foods we're trying to avoid on this protocol. Use a high-quality general probiotic like the Hyperbiotics® PRO-15, or see the full Supplements chapter for specific targeted strains.

Now, when it comes to antifungals, antimicrobials, and antibiotics, like neem, berberine, and oregano oil that are said to be effective at eliminating bacteria, I would proceed with caution.

Not all gut issues are the result of yeast, fungal, or bacterial overgrowth, and taking the supplements can actually do more harm than good and wipe out beneficial bacteria too. If you're interested in going down this route, and maybe think you are dealing with a fungal or bacterial overgrowth, *do not* try to take care of it at home by yourself with these natural methods. The overlap between these conditions is massive, and I've personally seen how treating them ineffectively based on random lists of symptoms found on the internet can lead to long-term gut damage. Just because they're "natural" antibiotics doesn't mean they won't touch the good guys too.

Seriously, if you think you have Candida, or SIBO, or something of the sort, go to see a doctor or a naturopath who is willing and able to do a stool sample to determine the real issue. In the absence of this event, it's my personal opinion that antifungals and antibacterials should be avoided – there's no need to overcomplicate things when you can get there with diet alone.

Only proceed to the next sections if you have been tested and know for certain what ailment you are dealing with, and make sure that all choices you make are done with a healthcare professional.

Anti-Fungal, Anti-Yeast, and Anti-Bacterial Diet Protocol

Just like any of the protocols, our first step here is going to be to minimize the causes of fungal, yeast, and bacterial overgrowth with our diet.

While all of these different types of gut overgrowth differ in severity, they have shockingly similar root causes. In the vast majority of cases, overgrowth is caused by eating refined carbohydrates (e.g. bread), yeast-heavy foods (e.g. beer), too many starches, too much sugar, or foods high in mold.

While there are differences between "Candida" and "SIBO" diets, they usually include foods that aren't typically safe for acne-prone skin regardless (the Candida diet typically allows for the consumption of many grains, for instance).

We're basically going to adopt the Clear Skin Diet Blueprint with a handful of extra caveats:

- Avoid all added sugars
- Avoid high-sugar fruits
- Avoid high-mold foods (anything aged, mushrooms, foods with vinegar, old or aged meat and seafood, bread, sauerkraut, very ripe avocados, some nuts and seeds)
- Avoid all dairy
- Avoid all starches, legumes, and grains (bread, wheat, beans of all variety, and even "safe" starches, including sweet potatoes, regular potatoes, carrots, yam, rice, yucca, etc.)
- Coffee, chocolate, cacao (and preferably tea, but tea is still a better alternative if you need to have caffeine)

So, what *can* you eat on an anti-fungal diet?

- Non-starchy vegetables
- Lower sugar fruit in moderate amounts (e.g. berries, lemons, limes, olives, non-ripe avocados)
- Either very fresh meat and seafood or meat and seafood that has recently been defrosted (you want to avoid aged or even slightly old meat and seafood due to mold issues that can exacerbate fungal overgrowth)
- Healthy fats: ghee, beef tallow, coconut oil, MCT oil, etc. (avoid butter for now)
- Low-mold nuts and seeds in moderate amounts (almonds, macadamias, sunflower seeds, flaxseed, coconuts)
- Most herbs and spices are fine (see Clear Skin Diet

Blueprint)

I can't give you a timeframe on this diet, because people experience improvement from symptoms at rapidly different times. As a rule of thumb, I would try and stick to this protocol for at least a month *before* adding any of the supplements and medicines below.

Supplement Protocol for SIBO

If you tested positive for SIBO and are looking for an alternative to prescription antibiotics, I recommend talking to your healthcare provider about the following:

- Oil of Oregano (two drops a day, or the recommended serving amount in capsule form)
- Berberine (two capsules, twice daily)
- Colloidal silver (take recommended dosage on bottle)
- A high-quality probiotic, like Hyperbiotics® PRO-15 or Skinesa®
- Caprylic acid (800mg twice a day)

These supplements are aimed at eliminating SIBO overgrowth while maintaining as much of the healthy gut microbiome as possible. It's typically recommended to use a protocol like this for at least a month to ensure complete remission.

Supplement Protocol for Candida and Other Fungal Overgrowth

If you tested positive for Candida *or* a form of fungal overgrowth like SIFO, and are looking for an alternative to prescription medications, I recommend talking to your healthcare provider about the following:

- Oil of Oregano (two drops a day, or recommended serving

amount in capsule form)
- Capric acid (take recommended amount in capsule or liquid form)
- Caprylic acid (take recommended amount in capsule or liquid form)
- A high-quality probiotic, like Hyperbiotics® PRO-15 or Skinesa®

These supplements are aimed at eliminating Candida overgrowth while maintaining as much of the healthy gut microbiome as possible. It's typically recommended to use a protocol like this for at least a month to ensure complete remission.

Chapter 18: Fungal Acne Protocol

Do you have stubborn acne or dandruff that won't seem to go away (even after trying other protocols)? Do you have flakes around your nose, chin, eyebrows, or scalp? Do you have pus-filled whiteheads, or itchy, red patches of skin?

If you answered yes to any of those questions, you might *not* be dealing with acne – you could have fungal acne, which occurs due to an overgrowth of a fungus called Malassezia.

Fungal acne looks and feels a lot like acne (with a greater emphasis on whiteheads and flakey, red patches of skin skin) but manifests itself in different ways. Thus, it needs to be eliminated in a similar but slightly nuanced way. Fungal acne is, well, a *fungal* infection, whereas regular acne is a *bacterial* infection.

From a clinical perspective, fungal "acne" is *not* technically even acne – it's a fungal condition called Malassezia folliculitis that just happens to *look* like acne. I'll continue to refer to Malassezia folliculitis as "fungal acne" for the time being, as it's a whole lot easier, but keep in mind that these are two separate diseases.

Furthermore, we have *significantly* less research on dietary strategies to combat facial dermatitis or Malassezia folliculitis, as "fungal acne" is a relatively new subject of study, all things considered. Still, fungal acne seems to be a modern epidemic, with more and more individuals realizing that it's not acne they struggle with, but Malassezia folliculitis.

For this reason, this protocol is going to be a bit different than the others, since we're essentially looking at a whole new disease here. The good news is that the very same root causes of acne, including insulin, inflammation, and gut dysbiosis, play a significant role in fungal acne, too.

How Do I know if I Have Fungal Acne or Regular Acne?

The largest difference between fungal acne and regular acne is in the visible appearance of the lesions, or the pimples. Do you have white, pus-filled pimples and redness around particular areas (nose and lips is very common)? Is it very itchy, and sometimes burning? Do you also struggle with dandruff, flakes around the eyebrows and nose, or another form of psoriasis or dermatitis? Then you're likely dealing with fungal acne.

On the other hand, if you mainly deal with blackheads, red bumps, or deep cysts (which are *not* pus-filed whiteheads), you're probably dealing with regular acne.

There is no sure-fire way to know if you're dealing with regular acne or fungal acne, but if you've had acne for a while and tried a bunch of different things, you may truly be dealing with a fungal issue rather than a bacterial one.

A quick image search of "malassezia folliculitis" or "fungal acne" will provide you with a plethora of good examples of fungal acne. For most people, it will be *very* obvious that they have fungal acne because their skin will look extremely similar to the images.

Fungal Acne 101

Malassezia, the fungi responsible for fungal acne, is naturally found on the skin. Everyone has Malassezia, and it's a lot like sebum oil in many regards - it's necessary and beneficial in small amounts, but problematic when it grows and spreads too rapidly. When the balance of Malassezia is thrown off on the skin or scalp, fungal infections and overgrowth can occur, leading to tons of different skin conditions, including fungal acne, seborrheic dermatitis (dandruff), psoriasis, and eczema. Basically, a fungal infection can cause just about every skin issue out there, so it's super important to keep Malassezia levels regulated and the skin microbiome healthy enough to handle Malassezia. Much like sebum oil, though, this is only part of the issue.

Individuals who have a compromised immune system, who have used large amounts of acne products in the past (especially steroid or retinol-based products), or who taken several rounds of prescription antibiotics are particularly suspectable to this fungal overgrowth that leads to what *seems* like acne.

Furthermore, just like bacterial acne, fungal acne isn't really a problem until an *inflammatory* response takes place. Everyone has Malassezia on the surface of their skin, but the puss-filled and protruding pimples, redness, and flakes that accompany fungal acne *only* take place when inflammation takes over. The body mistakes Malassezia for a threat and triggers an inflammatory response, leading to the appearance of fungal acne.

This might sound problematic, but for our purposes this is actually a pretty big advantage – throughout this book we've thoroughly studied the largest contributors to inflammation, including consumption of insulin-spiking foods, omega-6 fatty acids, and foods high in anti-nutrients. You already have *most* of the tools you need to beat fungal acne, but there are a few tweaks that will prove valuable in order to beat it.

What's Different About Treating Fungal Acne?

It could be years before we have research on the dietary triggers for fungal acne like we do with bacterial acne, but what we *do* have is a plethora of evidence that other forms of fungal skin conditions, including dermatitis, psoriasis, and eczema *can* be improved by taking certain dietary measures.

Fungal acne is a bit harder to treat than regular acne because we have considerably less evidence on what the internal, root causes of fungal acne really are. We know inflammation and an overactive immune system is a huge factor, but there very well may be other underlying issues that are triggering the outbreak.

In addition, many of the common foods that help kill acne bacteria may actually *contribute* to fungal overgrowth, including coconut oil (the lauric acid in coconut oil has been shown to feed Malassezia) and other high-saturated fat foods.

Furthermore, low-carb diets, including the ketogenic diet or carnivore diet *can* lead to certain nutritional deficiencies that make individuals more susceptible to fungal overgrowth.

For this reason, fungal acne requires a slightly different approach than the other types of acne we've discussed so far. Certain foods that are regularly safe for acne will have to be avoided, some nutrient-dense foods or supplements may need to be added, and topical adjustments may be necessary.

The Fungal Acne Diet

In order to minimize Malassezia overgrowth *and* decrease inflammation, we want to adopt an *anti-fungal* and anti-inflammatory diet for a period of time.

I'll outline two dietary protocols below: a protocol for mild-to-moderate fungal acne and a temporary protocol for severe fungal acne. Try starting with some of the changes in the Basic protocol before jumping into the Advanced protocol.

Basic Fungal Acne Diet Protocol

The Clear Skin Diet Protocol is already a great start for beating fungal acne, as it's naturally low in inflammation-causing foods. For the most part we'll be following the protocol with a few subtle additions:

- Avoid overconsumption of high-sugar fruits
- Avoid consuming fermented alcohol (beer, champagne, cider)
- Avoid consuming fermented foods (yogurt, kefir, kombucha, sauerkraut, etc.)
- Avoid high-mold foods (anything aged, mushrooms, foods with vinegar, old or aged meat and seafood, bread, sauerkraut, very ripe avocados, some nuts and seeds)
- Avoid dairy except ghee or grass-fed butter
- Avoid coconut oil, as the lauric acid may contribute to Malassezia overgrowth

Remember, these changes should be added *in addition to* the Clear Skin Diet Protocol. These are specific, targeted dietary actions that will limit fungus and yeast overgrowth that promotes fungal acne. Additionally, we will cover supplements that can help combat fungal acne in a subsequent section.

Advanced Fungal Acne Diet Protocol

If you've been struggling with fungal acne for a while and it's quite severe, you may want to jump into a protocol that eliminates or greatly minimizes yeast and fungus-producing foods. This includes:

- Avoid *all* added sugars
- Avoid high-sugar fruits
- Avoid *all* dairy except ghee
- Avoid all starches, legumes, and grains (bread, wheat, beans of all variety, and even "safe" starches, including sweet potatoes, regular potatoes, carrots, yam, rice, yucca, etc.)
- Avoid coffee, chocolate, cacao (and preferably tea, but tea is still a better alternative if you need to have caffeine)
- Avoid coconut oil (fine in most cases, but there is some research that shows coconut oil actually feeds the Malassezia, the fungus that causes fungal acne)

Here are the safe foods on The Advanced Fungal Acne Diet:

- Biotin and Riboflavin rich foods: organ meats, salmon, and egg yolks (avoid egg whites)
- Non-starchy vegetables
- Lower sugar fruit in moderate amounts (e.g. berries, lemons, limes, olives, non-ripe avocados)
- Either very fresh meat and seafood or meat and seafood that has recently been defrosted (you want to avoid aged or even slightly old meat and seafood due to mold issues that can exacerbate fungal overgrowth)
- Healthy fats: ghee, beef tallow, MCT oil, etc. (avoid butter and coconut oil for now)
- Low-mold nuts and seeds in moderate amounts (almonds, macadamias, sunflower seeds, flaxseed)
- Most herbs and spices are fine (see Clear Skin Diet Blueprint)

Again, this does *not* mean you can never eat these foods again. Our goal is to minimize fungus production while building up the gut microbiome.

Necessary Dietary Additions to Beat Fungal Acne: Foods High in B-Vitamins Riboflavin and Biotin

A lot folks looking to get clear skin will naturally transition to a lower carb, ketogenic, or carnivore diet. While this is an *amazing* switch to make when it comes to beating inflammation and bacterial acne, there is actually a pretty big nutritional pitfall that *can* occur when it comes to fungal acne: riboflavin and biotin deficiency.

Biotin and riboflavin are two vitamins that are used in fat absorption and utilization, particularly when in ketosis. These vitamins are involved in the process of allowing cells to utilize fat for energy. In simple terms, when our body goes to store or mobilize fat, these vitamins help with the process.

The more fat you consume, the higher the requirements of these two B-vitamins. Hopefully, you're starting to see why this can be an issue: in lower carb diets, carbohydrate consumption is typically replaced with higher consumption of fats, which, in turn, requires increased amounts of biotin and riboflavin. It's no surprise that one study found that low-carbohydrate diets seem to exacerbate biotin deficiency[90].

The problem is that both of these B-Vitamins are *crucial* for healthy, clear skin. Riboflavin is necessary for proper antioxidant functioning, collagen production, and hydration of the skin, all factors that play a role in how the skin reacts to Malassezia. Biotin is necessary for adequate for healthy, strong skin, hair and nails. Studies show that both biotin and riboflavin deficiency lead to a perfect breeding ground for fungal acne: dry, cracked, itchy and weak skin[91].

While transitioning to a lower carb diet is a great choice for *any* type of acne, fungal or not, you have to make sure that you're getting adequate biotin and riboflavin on lower carb diets to make up for the increase in fat intake, otherwise you're making yourself considerably more suspectable to fungal acne and dermatitis.

For this reason, consuming biotin and riboflavin rich foods, including egg yolks (avoid egg whites, as they bind to biotin and make it difficult to absorb), salmon, and organ meats like liver is crucial. A moderate serving of salmon, a few egg yolks, or a few ounces of liver per week is enough to do the trick.

If you *can't* obtain these food-based sources of B-Vitamins, refer to the supplementation strategy below.

Fungal Acne Supplements

There are many similarities between the supplements outlined in this section and the supplements outlined in the Clear Skin Protocol, but there are a handful of nutrients that are absolutely essential *if you're not getting them through dietary sources*. Here are several I would consider specifically to combat fungal acne.

Zinc

One study found that oral administration of zinc led to significant improvements in atopic dermatitis, a condition much like fungal acne[92]. Given zinc's role in combatting inflammation, it makes sense that it would improve the symptoms of fungal acne, in which an overactive immune system triggers an inflammatory response to the natural Malassezia fungi on the skin. Generally, folks will take around 30mg of zinc per day.

Biotin and Riboflavin

As we discussed, biotin and riboflavin are two nutrients in which deficiency is highly associated with dermatitis and fungal acne. If you can't get your biotin and riboflavin through food-based sources like liver, egg yolks, or wild-caught salmon, it is extremely advantageous to supplement with these b-vitamins, particularly if you're on a high-fat or ketogenic diet. 100mg of both biotin and riboflavin per day are common.

Anti-Fungal Supplements

In addition to giving yourself the nutrients necessary to combat inflammation and have healthy, strong skin, many individuals find simple anti-fungal supplements to go a long way in the fight to internally curing fungal acne. While I don't recommend taking antibiotics or even strong over-the-counter anti-fungal supplements like oregano oil for this purpose, there are a few supplements that many people I've worked with in the past found helpful, namely caprylic and capric acid.

You can buy caprylic and capric acid supplements, often in pill form (take about a gram a day of each), or you can buy MCT oil. The key is to make sure that the MCT oil does *not* contain lauric acid – lauric acid actually feeds Malassezia, which makes it problematic for fungal acne. This is why MCT oil, as opposed to coconut oil, is key.

I recommend using a high-quality probiotic, like Hyperbiotics® PRO-15, or the Skinesa® probiotic, alongside this protocol, as many people struggle with fungal acne due to prior antibiotic use.

This might seem a little light, especially compared to the other anti-fungal supplement protocols, but remember that too many antibiotics and antifungals, even "natural" ones, can destroy the good bacteria and fungi in tour gut, too.

Fungal Acne Topical Care

While I highly prefer to take an internal approach to acne, fungal acne is a bit unique in the fact that we don't have a wealth of research regarding its internal and dietary causes like we do with bacterial acne.

For this reason, I'll offer a handful of practical tips others claim to have helped eliminate fungal acne.

MCT Oil Cleanse

As we covered in the supplements area, MCT oil is loaded with capric and caprylic acid (make sure you don't buy MCT oil that contains lauric acid), which is a Malassezia-killing machine. Applying MCT oil to the skin topically is a surefire way to start combatting the fungal overgrowth and get your skin back to its natural state without drying out the skin or destroying the colonies of good bacteria that protect your skin.

As an added bonus, while coconut oil is comedogenic, meaning it can clog pores (which we all know can lead to acne infections), MCT oil is non-comedogenic and extremely moisturizing.

There's no blueprint on the perfect way to do an oil cleanse, but when I struggled with fungal acne and dandruff and used MCT oil to cure it, here was my rough regime:

- Once a day, massage a small layer of MCT oil around all parts of your face, neck, and scalp (if you have dandruff)
- Leave it on the skin for 5-15 minutes
- Wash your face with lukewarm water, and use a clean, ideally soft, microfiber cloth to wipe off the excess oil

That's it; it's really that simple.

Salt Rinses

Another easy fix for fungal acne is to incorporate salt rinses into your skincare routine. Salt is one of nature's most abundant antifungal compounds. A lot of folks on the GoodGlow blog and on other forums have experienced pretty profound results from incorporating salt rinses into their skincare routine (also useful for dandruff, dermatitis, and psoriasis).

Simply take 4 parts water to 1 part sea salt, Pink Himalayan salt, or Dead Sea salt, and rinse the face and scalp with the water. You can also spray the face or submerge the face in salt water. Let it sit for a few minutes, and then rinse off.

Sulfur

Sulfur is an extremely powerful anti-fungal compound that luckily is relatively safe on the skin overall. Compared to something like benzoyl peroxide, sulfur does less to eliminate bacteria and far more to eliminate yeast and fungi on the skin, which makes it ideal for fungal acne.

You can get precipitated sulfur soap or sulfur ointment and use it once or twice a day. Look for 10% sulfur content and as few added ingredients as possible.

Zinc

Applying zinc topically to the skin is another popular strategy to combat fungal acne. Like sulfur, there are two ways to go about this: zinc soap or zinc cream.

In the case of zinc soap, again, look for something with minimum added ingredients (to avoid anything that could potentially feed yeast and fungi) and 2% pyrithione zinc.

In the case of cream, look for "zinc oxide" (oftentimes sold as baby powder) with the fewest number of added ingredients.

Nothing (Caveman Protocol)

At its core, fungal acne occurs because of the body's inability to tolerate a naturally occurring fungi on the surface of the skin. In many cases, this is due to a skin microbiome that has been damaged after years of attempting to treat acne. For this reason, many individuals find relief from fungal acne by allowing their skin to recover and adopting a "caveman" protocol. Simply washing their face with water once or twice a day allows the skin's beneficial bacteria to start building up again, which play a role in combatting both fungal overgrowth and the inflammation that leads to fungal acne.

Chapter 19: Carnivore Protocol

The carnivore diet consists of eating only animal-based foods. It is extremely low in carbohydrates, and because it includes no plant foods, the biggest culprits for inflammation-driven acne (lectins, phytate, saponins, etc.) are avoided. That means it sidesteps many of the largest triggers for acne completely.

Still, it is challenging to adhere to, and for this reason I don't necessarily recommend adopting the diet unless you have to, or specifically want to. Some people find it rather extreme, but the effects related to acne can be profound because, if done properly, it essentially eliminates all three root causes of acne.

What Can you Eat on the Carnivore Protocol?

The carnivore diet generally is defined as eating only foods from the "animal kingdom". What's considered "carnivore" can differ from person to person. What just about every carnivore can agree on is that meat and seafood are okay, including (but not limited to):

- Beef
- Lamb
- Bison
- Elk
- Sheep
- Pork
- Chicken
- Salmon
- Sardines

- Tuna
- Clams
- Etc.

In addition, some carnivores include foods that come from animals, like butter, milk, cheese, or eggs. Others even include coffee and tea.

While these additions might not help individuals doing the carnivore diet to lose weight, if undertaking this protocol in an attempt to get rid of acne, I recommend *avoiding* these added foods and sticking solely to meat and seafood.

A pure carnivore diet consisting of only meat, seafood, water, and salt (no dairy, no egg whites) is probably the safest diet out there when it comes to acne:

- By eliminating plant foods, you minimize the consumption of antinutrients that can damage the gut and cause inflammation and acne
- By eliminating foods with carbohydrates (meat and seafood have practically no carbs), you reduce the amount of insulin your body releases and stop hormonal acne
- Meat intolerance is extremely rare, so you're unlikely to trigger digestive issues

A common question regarding the carnivore diet is, "Won't I get nutritional deficiencies?" and the simple answer is no; or at least it's unlikely, *especially* if you're eating organ meats. The section below will explain more of this, but in reality, organ meats are some of the best sources of acne-fighting nutrients on the planet and contain these nutrients in bioavailable forms that our bodies crave.

Still, the carnivore diet is extremely *new*. By virtue of the fact that we don't have much research on it, I can't sit here and advocate that anyone tries it – only that you may want to consider it if you have attempted other methods and are still struggling. It has worked for countless individuals, but we honestly don't know the long-term positive or negative side-effects of the diet.

Here's how to optimize the carnivore diet for beating acne.

1. Eat mostly red meat or fatty fish when you're hungry, and stop when you're full

When it comes to nutritionally dense and easily digestible meat, ruminants top the chart. Ruminants include beef, goat, sheep, and bison. While you can eat any type of meat you want, I've found that most carnivores get the majority of their calories from those 4 nutrient-dense meats. Wild-caught fatty fish, like salmon or mackerel, are also great sources of nutrition.

Furthermore, while you can incorporate intermittent fasting with the carnivore diet, it's not a requirement. It is typical to eat anywhere from 1.5 to 3 pounds of meat per day.

2. Don't worry about organic/free-range meat (but buy free range eggs and wild-caught fish)

Dr. Shawn Baker, an avid carnivore, did some research regarding the nutrient profile of grass-fed, organic beef compared to conventional factory-farmed beef and found little evidence of huge nutritional differences. While I would still prefer organic, grass-fed meat over conventional meat, the differences in fatty acid profiles were negligible.

With that being said, eggs and fish are a different story – conventional eggs contain more omega-6 fatty acids than free-range eggs by a considerable amount, and contain fewer nutrients. Wild-caught fish is a great source of omega-3 fatty acids, whereas farmed fish, especially salmon, is actually high enough in omega-6 fatty acids that the benefits from the omega-3s will be significantly diminished.

If you can't afford wild-caught fish (sardines are by far the cheapest and almost always wild-caught) consider supplementing with a wild-caught fish or krill oil supplement.

3. Add organ meats

As we covered in the diet section, organ meats are amazing for your overall health and your skin. For acne, liver is definitely the most powerful organ meat thanks to its extremely high vitamin A content. If you want to supercharge your carnivore diet, eat organ meat at least once a week - especially liver, if you can get your hands on it.

Furthermore, organ meats contain two *essential* B-Vitamins that you *need* on the carnivore diet: biotin and riboflavin.

Both biotin and riboflavin are used in the process of transporting and storing fat – something that your body will have to do quite frequently on the carnivore diet due to the lack of carbohydrates. The more fat you eat, the higher your body's requirement for riboflavin and biotin.

Without biotin and riboflavin, your body can't provide the lipids necessary for your skin to be protected and healthy – it becomes read, dry, cracked, and irritated, which makes it the perfect breeding ground for fungal acne.

You can view the full Fungal Acne Protocol for more details, but a lot of times when individuals on the carnivore diet struggle to achieve clear skin, it's *not* due to bacterial acne but rather yeast and fungi overgrowth on the skin. The carnivore diet will go a long way in decreasing the inflammation that accompanies this overgrowth, but if you are on the carnivore diet and struggle with dandruff or dermatitis, consider increasing these B-Vitamins by consuming organ meats (ideal), egg yolks, or salmon at least once a week.

I would go as far as saying that if you *can't* add organ meats, either in the form of real organs or desiccated organ supplements, that you should possibly reconsider the carnivore diet for acne.

4. Add wild-caught fatty fish

Wild-caught, fatty fish, like salmon, mackerel, and sardines, are an amazing source of omega-3 fatty acids that help prevent inflammatory acne. Unfortunately, farmed fish contain high amounts of inflammatory omega-6 fatty acids and can contain compounds that exacerbate acne triggers in some individuals. If you can, eat wild-caught fatty fish once a week (make sure that if it's salmon you're eating the skin, where most of the omega-3s are).

5. Cut out all dairy except ghee (and possibly butter)

This isn't a requirement, as many carnivores consider dairy fair-game, but if you want the best results for acne it's best to cut out dairy, at least for a period of time. With the notable exception of ghee (and butter, if you can tolerate it), dairy oftentimes contains and causes the release of acne-causing hormones, can trigger inflammation, and can damage the gut. It's often better to just avoid it.

6. Consider cutting out egg whites

On top of dairy, you may also want to cut out eggs, and more particularly the whites. While egg yolks are a great source of fat-soluble vitamins and healthy fats, egg whites are notoriously common digestive disruptors. Many people simply can't handle egg whites, and their skin ends up breaking out.

7. Watch out for chicken and pork

Chicken and pork are almost always fine, but some people have issues with both of these meats when it comes to acne. In the case of chicken, it's oftentimes extremely high in omega-6 fatty acids, which can cause inflammation. This is especially true in the case of factory-farmed dark meat chicken or chicken skin.

In the case of pork, some people seem to have very intense blood sugar reactions to pork, which causes them to produce a bunch of insulin that causes acne. That's why, just like any other protocol, the key is to experiment with what meat works for you. You might find chicken works *better* than other meat.

8. Don't go overboard on the protein

This is just from personal experience, but too much protein and not enough fat can cause me to break out. I know, it's tempting to eat 2 pounds of sirloin steak every day, but I personally found my energy and my skin doing best on fattier cuts of meat cooked in saturated fat like beef tallow or grass-fed ghee. Ribeye, chuck, lamb shoulder and legs, chicken thighs and wings, and fatty fish like salmon are all great sources of healthy fats and adequate amounts of protein.

9. Give it time

My skin definitely improved on the carnivore diet, but it took some time. If there's anything I've learned from switching my diet up a lot over the last four or five years, it's that acne *almost* always gets worse before it gets better. For starters, you'll probably find yourself losing fat on the carnivore diet. Waste by-products are stored in fat, and they can be released through the skin. You also may find yourself stressed out or missing some of your favorite foods – this can cause acne too.

Give it at least 30 days, and I think you'll find that the carnivore diet is great for your skin. Be patient, tweak it if you have to, and above all else, listen to your body.

Sample day of eating

A lot of folks wonder – what the heck do you eat in a day on the carnivore diet? My number one piece of advice here is to listen to your body. I do far, far better with a single large meal in a day. When I'm in "carnivore" mode, I eat upwards of two and a half pounds of meat over the course of an hour or maybe an hour and a half. A more traditional carnivore diet might look like this:

Breakfast:

- 2 eggs, 4 slices of bacon (if you can tolerate pork and eggs)
- 12oz. pound of ground beef (if you can't tolerate pork and eggs)
- Lunch/snack:
- A few soft-boiled eggs yolks
- 8oz. of lamb shoulder
- Dinner:
- 1 pound of fatty red meat slathered in ghee

Summary: Carnivore Protocol

I think that the carnivore protocol probably isn't necessary for the vast majority of people, but one thing I will say as someone who tried it for a while is that you may actually be surprised by how well it suits you. A lot of folks start the carnivore protocol to get rid of acne and stay with it because of how much better they feel. If you want a little more flexibility, check out the Gut Protocol, which is still a largely animal-based diet with a few of the safest additions.

Chapter 20: Plant-Based Protocol

A vegetarian diet consists of eating only plant-based foods, with the notable exceptions of eggs and sometimes dairy and honey. A vegan diet consists of abstaining from all foods that are animal-based, which means eggs, dairy, and honey are off the table. Plant-based diets of this sort can cause issues for acne because they are typically higher in carbs and antinutrients than other diets; however, by avoiding insulin-spiking foods, industrial oils and plants with high amounts of antinutrients, most of these issues can be avoided.

There are plenty of reasons you might want to go vegetarian or vegan, whether it's for ethical, social, or health-related reasons. While you certainly don't have to go vegetarian for clear skin (in fact, if your *only* goal is clear skin, I'd actually recommend against it), many people would prefer to make the switch to plant-based.

The downside is that there are a *lot* of pitfalls that can trip people up when switching to a vegetarian diet. The good news is that regardless of your choice to be a carnivore, omnivore, or herbivore, achieving clear skin is possible with the right strategy.

Note: This protocol is strictly speaking a <u>vegetarian</u> protocol, meaning that I will be including eggs in the diet. If you would like to modify this diet to fit a vegan lifestyle, simply remove eggs.

1. Avoid excessive carbohydrate consumption

Many vegetarian or vegan diets are high in carbs simply because they exclude animal-based food, which is almost exclusively carbohydrate-free. Vegetarians oftentimes replace animal protein with carb-rich plant foods, which is fine if you're super active, but problematic if they're your *only* source of nutrients. Many fresh fruits contain fiber that offset their sugar content, but still, it can add up. Make sure that your vegetarian diet contains plenty of healthy, *fatty*, plant-based food:

- Egg yolks (if vegetarian)
- Macadamia nuts (and other nuts, if you tolerate them)
- Avocados, avocado oil
- Coconut, coconut oil
- Olives, olive oil

Make sure you steer clear of the following insulin-spiking, nutritionally void foods:

- Fruit juice
- Soda
- White potatoes (in excess)
- Dates, bananas, raisins, and watermelon (in excess)

Keep your consumption of safe starches to a minimum – try not to overindulge in white rice, yam, sweet potatoes, pumpkins, or cassava, as they all have a relatively high glycemic index.

2. Stay clear of grains, legumes, and unsafe starches

By now you definitely have a grasp of why the lectins and other antinutrients found in grains, legumes, and unsafe starches are problematic for individuals with acne-prone skin. They wreak havoc on our digestive system and can cause chronic inflammation.

Vegetarian diets are oftentimes high in foods with these antinutrients, so it's important to try and keep the following foods to a minimum, or try eliminating them for a period of time before reintroducing them:

- Corn, corn-based products (chips, tortillas, popcorn, etc.)
- Wheat (bread, pasta, pastries, etc.)
- Buckwheat, quinoa, and oats (safter than bread, but make sure you test them)
- Grain-based products (cereal, oatmeal, many nutritional/granola bars)
- Beans and legumes, unless properly soaked and cooked (make sure you test them)
- Peanuts
- Beer
- Non-white rice may cause grain-like issues as well
- Fake meat (almost always contains soybeans)
- Tofu (soybean)

3. Avoid inflammation-causing vegetable oils

One problem you frequently run into on a vegan or vegetarian diet is that in the absence of healthy animal fats, food manufacturers and restaurants will often use industrial vegetable oils loaded with omega-6 fatty acids (remember, omega-6 is an inflammatory fatty acid that can trigger acne).

While it's technically vegan, your body simply isn't capable of breaking down these inflammatory oils. Many of them contain ten to twenty times the amount of omega-6 than healthier alternatives, like avocado, olive, or coconut oil.

On a vegetarian diet, make sure you avoid the following oils, **as well as any products that contain these oils**:

- Safflower oil
- Sunflower oil
- Canola oil

- Peanut oil
- Soy oil
- Cottonseed oil
- Corn oil
- Vegetable oil (combination of oils)
- Flaxseed oil
- Margarine

Unfortunately, tons of vegan and plant-based foods are *loaded* with these oils, because they're cheap and easy to manufacture. Instead, opt for these vegetarian oils and fats:

- Ghee (if vegetarian)
- Coconut oil (preferably virgin, organic)
- Extra-virgin olive oil
- Avocado oil
- Macadamia nut oil
- Cacao butter
- Palm oil

4. Supplement with an algae-based Omega-3

The only common foods that are truly high in usable DHA and EPA omega-3 are all animal based: fatty fish and organ meats. Even if you're eating tons of walnuts, or other foods high in omega-3s, you'll be consuming ALA omega-3 (alongside tons of omega-6s to cancel any benefit out), which is extremely inefficient for the body to process.

Fortunately, plant-based algae omega-3 has been shown to be just as bioavailable, and sometimes more bioavailable, than non-vegan fish oil supplements (I actually take algae omega-3 personally, and I by no means eat a purely plant-based diet). I take roughly 700 mg of algae omega-3 per day, containing 195mg of EPA and 390mg of DHA (I sometimes will take cod liver supplements as well).

5. Limit high-phytate foods and supplement with zinc

When it comes to acne-fighting nutrients, it's hard to beat zinc. One study found that zinc went head-to-head with dangerous prescription antibiotics when it comes to its power for decreasing acne over a three-month period (without all the negative damage to the gut microbiome)[93]. Unfortunately, many common foods on plant-based diets inhibit the absorption of zinc due to their phytate content, and many of the best sources of zinc come from the animal kingdom (clams, oysters, crabs, lamb, beef, etc.).

So, our strategy needs to be twofold. First, we need to limit plant-based foods which contain large amounts phytates that prevent us from absorbing zinc, including:

- Grains (wheat, corn, rye, etc.)
- Most legumes – soy, pinto, kidney, navy beans, peanuts, lentils
- Some nuts – almonds, hazelnuts, brazil nuts, cashews
- Potatoes
- Uncooked spinach, chard, kale
- Dark chocolate

In addition to limiting high-phytate foods (you don't need to eliminate them – phytate may actually be *good* in moderate doses), you'll likely want to take a zinc supplement as well. Most of the best sources of zinc on a vegan diet, like lentils, contain phytates that prevent the zinc from being absorbed. So, while you're getting zinc on paper, in reality your body can't absorb any of it.

For that reason, it may be useful to supplement with zinc. When I was on a plant-heavy diet, I used 30mg of Zinc Picolinate from Thorne Research daily.

6. Eat foods high in vitamin A with a skin-safe fat or oil

When it comes to nutrients that fight acne, vitamin A is right alongside zinc when it comes to essential nutrients for clear skin. It reduces the amount of pore-clogging oil our skin produces, it improves wound healing and can help acne scars heal faster, it protects the skin from acne-causing free radicals, and it reduces inflammation.

While it's a common belief that vegetables are high in vitamin A, that's only part of the story. Vegetables are high in vitamin A, but they're high in what's called beta carotene, a form of vitamin A that needs to be converted into retinol in order to be used by the body.

In some cases, only a fraction of beta carotene found in plants actually gets converted into retinol. Some people are deficient in vitamin A despite eating foods with tons of beta carotene. That's also why you can't trust a nutrition label when it says a vegetable has 300% of your daily vitamin A.

Luckily, you can increase the absorption of beta carotene by doing two simple things: lightly cooking your vegetables and consuming cooked vegetables with a skin-friendly fat, like olive oil, coconut oil, or avocado oil.

Vitamin A is a fat-soluble vitamin, so either lightly sauteing your veggies in a skin-safe fat or oil or eating them alongside a saturated fat will greatly increase the amount of beta carotene that actually gets converted into usable, retinol vitamin A.

7. Stop eating soy and products with soy

Soy often becomes a staple when people switch to a plant-based diet, which can be a real disaster for acne-prone skin. Worse yet, soy is in tons of vegan products, including tofu, meatless burgers or meat alternatives, protein powder, and plant-based milk.

As we discussed in the diet section, there are some *huge* downsides to soy and soy-based products: they contain antinutrients (lectins and phytic acid) which prevent the body from absorbing acne-fighting nutrients, they disrupt your hormones, and in the case of soybean oil, it's high in inflammation-causing omega-6.

8. Be careful what's in your protein powder

Many plant-based protein powders are made out of pea, soy, or wheat-based protein, which can be harmful for acne. The reason for this is pretty straightforward: peas, soybeans, and wheat all contain lectins and phytic acid, and so do their protein-powder byproducts. If you're struggling with acne on a vegetarian diet, try cutting out the protein powder and see what happens. In general, I'm not a huge fan of protein powders for clear skin, regardless of whether or not they're plant-based.

9. Avoid soy, oat, hemp, and flaxseed milk (use coconut, macadamia, almond, or cashew milk instead)

Dairy milk is, admittedly, a disaster for acne – so when you switch a vegetarian diet, you might think you're in the clear when it comes to plant-based milk substitutes, right?

Nope. *Most* plant-based milk alternatives are a nightmare for acne. I've covered this in further detail in the Diet section, but for now, it's sufficient to say that coconut milk and macadamia milk are *by far* your best options, followed by cashew or almond milk if you can tolerate it.

Sample Plant-Based Clear Skin Diet

This is a list of just some of my favorite plant-based foods for clear skin – you don't have to stick exactly to this, but it's a decent starting place.

Healthy fats:

- Avocados
- Avocado oil
- Olive oil
- Coconut oil
- Macadamia nuts
- Almonds, cashews, pistachios, pecans, walnuts, brazil nuts (in moderation)

Vegetables:

A wide variety of vegetables, ideally cooked lightly and served with olive or avocado oil

Fruits:

All fresh, whole fruits (no dried fruits or fruit juice) eaten in moderation to avoid insulin spikes

Safe starches:

- White rice, yam, sweet potatoes, pumpkins, or cassava, all eaten in moderation
- White potatoes, in moderation, if tolerated

Other:

- Properly soaked and fully cooked legumes on occasion (lentils and chickpeas are safest)
- Tea, coffee, kombucha, and coconut water are all okay, assuming you tolerate them

Chapter 21: Thyroid Protocol

A lot of folks struggling with acne also have a thyroid disorder. In fact, it's so common that it's worth making a separate protocol for it, as some of the dietary tactics in the other protocols don't apply if you're dealing with a thyroid disorder. This can lead to a lot of frustration – "I've tried everything, why isn't this working!" Well, it may be due to your thyroid, especially if you're a woman and have struggled with cystic acne in the past.

Before we get there, we need to cover some of the basics about what the thyroid is and why it may be behind your acne.

Thyroid Health 101

The thyroid is a gland near your neck that has the important job of regulating your organs. It helps make sure you're energized and functioning throughout the day, and is one of the single most important glands in your entire body. Some of the thyroid's responsibilities include the regulation of digestion, heart function, mood, brain function, and metabolism.

In order to regulate all these processes, the thyroid secretes various thyroid *hormones*. These hormones, just like any other hormone, aren't necessarily good or bad – in the right amount, they are great! Too much and you can have anxiety, irritability, and mood swings. Too little and you can have chronic fatigue, dry skin, weakness, and, you guessed it, cystic acne.

While an overactive thyroid (called *hyper*thyroidism) is no walk in the park, if you're dealing with a thyroid-related acne issue it's probably due to an underactive thyroid, which is called *hypo*thyroidism. Rates of acne in women with thyroid issues are considerably higher than in individuals without thyroid issues[94], and it seems like they're becoming more and more common every year.

The Link Between Hypothyroidism and Acne

On a broader scale, it's no surprise that an unhealthy thyroid could cause acne. It impacts how our body handles nearly *everything*, and acne, being impacted by just about everything from our digestion to our sleep, will obviously worsen if our thyroid isn't in check. If we're not healthy in general, we can't expect our skin to be at its best. But more specifically, hypothyroidism comes with a unique set of issues that makes it problematic for those of us who deal with acne:

- An underactive thyroid lead to decreased levels of progesterone, which leads to *increased* estrogen levels. Too much estrogen can be a huge cause of hormonal acne, *especially* cystic acne
- A common symptom of hypothyroidism is dry, flakey skin, which can lead to clogged pores and weak, damaged skin
- Most importantly, a weakened immune system makes you less capable of handling oxidative stress and dealing with inflammatory acne[95]

This last point is what we're going to focus on for the most part. It's estimated that an astounding 90% of all individuals suffering from hypothyroidism have a specific condition called Hashimoto's Disease[96], which is an autoimmune disease.

We've already discussed autoimmune conditions in depth, but the key thing to remember is that autoimmune conditions mistake trivial, everyday processes as threats. Certain foods, drinks, and environmental factors that a healthy immune system could handle just fine turn into events that trigger acne-causing inflammation.

The good news is that this isn't incurable - it's just going to be a bit more challenging than treating a thyroid issue all by itself. The protocol you adopt will have to not only improve thyroid health (potentially using iodine, zinc, vitamin D, or prescribed medication), but also *avoid* triggering the inflammatory response that is caused by Hashimoto's.

How to know if you have hypothyroidism

If you struggle with acne, you're not crazy for thinking you might have a thyroid disorder – it's particularly common with women, and rates of thyroid disorders are much higher among people with adult acne, especially cystic acne. In fact, it's estimated that between 5 and 10% of the adult population struggle with hypothyroidism[97]. The only way to know for sure is to see a doctor and get a thyroid panel done. The following list of symptoms and signs is a good indicator for whether or not you should consider getting a thyroid panel:

- Constantly feeling cold
- Tiredness and fatigue, muscle weakness
- Depression
- Constipation
- Dry or flakey skin
- Slowed heart rate
- Stiff and painful joints
- Dry, thinning hair and hair loss
- Impaired memory
- Fertility difficulties or menstrual changes
- Puffy, sensitive face

Again, these symptoms don't replace a thyroid panel, but as someone who has been diagnosed with hypothyroidism, they're pretty spot on. Feeling cold, tired, and weak, were my most common symptoms, alongside dry hair, skin, and nails.

The Protocol Thyroid Acne Protocol

This protocol is great for anyone who has hypothyroidism or Hashimoto's. Even if you don't have Hashimoto's, if you struggle with acne and have an underactive thyroid, the odds are good that you would benefit by eating fewer inflammatory foods and adopting an autoimmune-friendly regimen.

This is *not* a substitute for thyroid hormone treatment or medical intervention. This should be seen as a way to mitigate and minimize the acne created by a thyroid disorder.

1. To Improve Thyroid Health: Iodine

Iodine is absolutely crucial for a properly functioning thyroid. Without enough iodine, your thyroid can't produce enough thyroid hormone to regulate processes like digestion, brain function, and muscle functioning, which is why if you have an underactive thyroid, you may feel tired or lethargic all the time. But *too much* iodine and you can actually cause hyperthyroidism. Many people find that all they needed to fix their thyroid issue was to cut out fluoride (usually from tea) and increase iodine consumption.

The highest food-based sources of iodine are kelp and seaweed, which, if you can get your hands on them, are great for other reasons too:

- May reduce oxidative stress and acne-causing inflammation[98]
- Lower levels of insulin, an acne-causing hormone typically triggered after meals containing large amounts of carbohydrates (it's why you tend to break out after a sugary meal)[99]
- May act as an antioxidant and help protect the skin from air pollution and UV damage[100]
- Kelp also contains vitamin K, an essential fat-soluble

vitamin for skin health

If you can't get seaweed, an iodine supplement will work just fine too – in fact, many iodine supplements have kelp as the primary ingredient, which means the iodine will be bioavailable and contain some of the nutrients kelp has to offer.

2. Eat a low-inflammation diet

Autoimmune disorders like Hashimoto's thrive on diets that are high in inflammatory compounds: gluten, sugar, and processed foods all trigger large autoimmune responses. Diets high in refined carbohydrates (breads, pasta, pizza, pastries, etc.) have been linked to hypothyroidism as well, while diets low in carbs may be better for hypothyroidism[101]. To avoid this, stick to the "safe" foods in the Diet section of this book, or the Clear Skin Diet Blueprint Protocol, both of which are low in inflammatory foods.

3. Consider an anti-inflammatory diet or supplement

Avoiding inflammatory foods is certainly the first step, but you might want to consider adding anti-inflammatory foods to your arsenal as well, which can help *prevent* autoimmune-driven inflammation from occurring. Increasing your omega-3 fatty either through eating fatty fish (salmon, sardines, mackerel), omega-3 supplements (algae, fish oil, krill oil, cod liver oil), or organ meats can be helpful.

4. Cut out tea

If you drink green, black, or oolong tea, I would recommend cutting it out for a period of time. This is due to the high fluoride content of tea, which contributes to hypothyroidism. If you must drink tea, drink white tea, which has about 1/3 the amount of fluoride as green or black tea. Still, if you can, cut out all tea for a period of time to see how you respond. If you need that caffeine in the morning to wake up (I sure know I do some days!), I recommend using an herbal tea and combining it with a caffeine powder or capsule. Coffee can also be problematic for autoimmune disorders, so I wouldn't necessarily just stop drinking tea, but instead stop drinking caffeinated tea.

5. Limit fluoride elsewhere

While tea is the biggest culprit of high fluoride intake for most people, there are other sources too. Here are a few drinks that contain high amounts of fluoride:

- Tap water (buy spring water, or purchase an alkaline water filter, which will remove around 80% of the fluoride)
- Wine
- Soda
- Fruit Juice

Switching to a non-fluorinated toothpaste can make a big difference too.

6. Consider Zinc and Vitamin D

We already know how important zinc and vitamin D are for fighting the root causes of acne:

- Preventing inflammation
- Improving digestion
- Promoting healthy sleep
- Increasing nutrient absorption

In addition, both zinc[102] and vitamin D[103] deficiencies are linked to higher rates of hypothyroidism. Supplementing with zinc, or cutting out foods high in phytates (legumes, grains, spinach, chard, peanuts, almonds, dark chocolate, etc.) and other antinutrients that prevent zinc from being absorbed may improve hypothyroidism.

7. Undereating/Fasting

Being in a caloric deficit (e.g. not eating enough), can also cause hypothyroidism. Individuals attempting to lose weight will oftentimes find themselves with thyroid issues if they try to do so too rapidly.

If you have thyroid issues and practice intermittent fasting, you may want to consider changing your fasting schedule or eating more during your meals. While intermittent fasting isn't directly linked to hypothyroidism, I know that I don't eat as much when I'm on a fasting routine. For quite some time, I had thyroid issues because I was undereating and underweight while practicing intermittent fasting. I really liked intermittent fasting, so instead of changing my schedule, I just made sure that I was eating enough at every meal. This, along with the supplements above, made a world of difference for my energy, mood, and thyroid.

Closing Thoughts

The journey doesn't end here – this is just the beginning.

Most diet, nutrition, or health-focused books end rather abruptly. They dump the information on your lap and say, "great, now go make it happen"! The unfortunate truth is that *most people* who read a book on weight loss, or diet, or fasting rarely incorporate the lessons from the book. This isn't the fault of the readers, nor necessarily the author, but rather a disconnect about expectations and goals. Throughout this book, I've done my best to empower you by giving you the *tools* you need to make excellent decisions for clear skin. My goal was not to give you a list of things to eat and things to avoid, but rather to explain the science behind *why* certain foods, supplements, or lifestyle choices are behind your acne and what *you* can do about it.

This might sound nerdy, but if you're like me, after reading this book and learning about all this stuff, you're probably pretty excited. You're excited to have found a method of achieving clear skin that doesn't revolve around an endless cycle of expensive cleansers and creams. You're excited to start making the steps towards clear skin. You're ready to start looking better and feelings better. My advice to you is simple: start now, start small, and be patient.

Starting now is absolutely crucial. *Use* this motivation that you feel right now because it *won't* last forever. This information is exciting, its fresh, and it's actionable. *Now* is the time to start making changes. Not next week, not after your next vacation, not after you finish a crazy work deadline, right *now*, today.

Starting small is just as important. Some people find that

making sweeping, drastic life changes is the only way they make real, lasting impact – they have to go all-out to make a change. For me, and for most of the GoodGlow readers I've helped over the years, this is *not* the case. The simple fact of the matter is that if you don't want to do this, it's not going to work. Instead of going for a 7-day fast off the rip, start by skipping a meal once or twice a week. Instead of cutting out caffeine cold turkey, scale back and wean off of it over the next few months. Instead of jumping into the Carnivore Protocol, maybe start with the Diet Blueprint protocol. Just because you start small doesn't mean you won't get big results – *take it one day at a time.*

Finally, being patient is absolutely crucial. While it's likely that you'll see results within a few weeks, this is *not* an overnight fix. Acne is something that developers over *years*, and it's going to take time to correct it. There will be setbacks, failures, and frustration. This is all part of the process. You need to ask yourself which frustration you would rather have: being frustrated at spending hundreds, if not thousands of dollars covering up the symptoms of acne with cleansers and creams, or being frustrated at the minor step-backs you'll inevitably face on the road to clear skin from within.

You will get through this, and the sooner you start tackling acne internally, the sooner you'll never have to worry about topical products again.

Resources to Use *Right Now*

While this book is fresh in your mind, I recommend utilizing a few free resources we've made to get started. All of these free resources were made to help you make the shift from "learning" to "doing" ...

The GoodGlow Diet Blueprint is a one-page sheet summarizing the Diet Blueprint Protocol. You can download it for free at: goodglow.co/blueprint

The GoodGlow Shopping Guide contains three simple guides for clear skin: a list of ingredients to avoid for clear skin, a guide to buying organic vs. conventional food for clear skin, and a list of simple grocery shopping tips. You can download it for free at goodglow.co/shopping-guide

We will be continuing the discussion on goodglow.co with new articles and videos related to clear skin from within.

Remember, the time to get started is *right now*.

About the Author

Sam Wood is founder of GoodGlow.co, an online resource for achieving permanently clear skin without the use of damaging acne products. Sam spent his early years struggling with acne. It took a toll on him not just physically, but emotionally and socially. After spending thousands of dollars on acne products only to find his acne coming back worse than ever, Sam began researching the link between various internal conditions and acne.

The research was clear: while acne appears on the surface of the skin, the root causes of acne are the result of diet and other internal factors. Using himself as a test subject, Sam experimented with different diets, supplements, and intermittent fasting. For the first (and only) time in his life, he found relief from acne. Frustrated by the lack of existing resources for achieving clear skin from within, Sam began researching nutritional science and started GoodGlow.co, a blog that has helped over 500,000 readers get started on the journey towards clear skin from within. You can reach Sam at info@goodglow.co.

Bibliography

[1] Bhate, K., & Williams, H. C. (2013). Epidemiology of acne vulgaris. *British Journal of Dermatology*, *168*(3), 474–485. https://doi.org/10.1111/bjd.12149

[2] Cordain, L., Lindeberg, S., Hurtado, M., Hill, K., Eaton, S. B., & Brand-Miller, J. (2002). Acne vulgaris: A disease of western civilization. *Archives of Dermatology*, *138*(12), 1584–1590. https://doi.org/10.1001/archderm.138.12.1584

[3] Kalvaitis, K. (2007, February 1). Generational decline in testosterone levels observed. Retrieved February 2, 2021, from Endocrine today website: https://www.healio.com/news/endocrinology/20120325/generational-decline-in-testosterone-levels-observed

[4] New CDC report: More than 100 million Americans have diabetes or prediabetes | CDC Online Newsroom | CDC. (2017, July 18). Retrieved February 2, 2021, from CDC Newsroom website: https://www.cdc.gov/media/releases/2017/p0718-diabetes-report.html

[5] Cappel, M., Mauger, D., & Thiboutot, D. (2005). Correlation between serum levels of insulin-like growth factor 1, dehydroepiandrosterone sulfate, and dihydrotestosterone and acne lesion counts in adult women. *Archives of Dermatology*, *141*(3), 333–338. https://doi.org/10.1001/archderm.141.3.333

[6] Emiroğlu, N., Cengiz, F. P., & Kemeriz, F. (2015). Insulin resistance in severe acne vulgaris. *Advances in Dermatology and Allergology*, *4*(4), 281–285. https://doi.org/10.5114/pdia.2015.53047/

[7] Bosma-Den Boer, M. M., Van Wetten, M. L., & Pruimboom, L. (2012). Chronic inflammatory diseases are stimulated by current lifestyle: How diet, stress levels and medication prevent our body from recovering. *Nutrition and Metabolism*, Vol. 9, p. 32. https://doi.org/10.1186/1743-7075-9-32

[8] Kris-Etherton, P. M., Taylor, D. S., Yu-Poth, S., Huth, P., Moriarty, K., Fishell, V., ... Etherton, T. D. (2000). Polyunsaturated fatty acids in the food chain in the United States. *American Journal of Clinical Nutrition*, *71*(1 SUPPL.), 179S-188S. https://doi.org/10.1093/ajcn/71.1.179s

[9] Simopoulos, A. P. (2002). The importance of the ratio of omega-6/omega-3 essential fatty acids. *Biomedicine and Pharmacotherapy*, *56*(8), 365–379. https://doi.org/10.1016/S0753-3322(02)00253-6

[10] Lobionda, S., Sittipo, P., Kwon, H. Y., & Lee, Y. K. (2019, August 1). The role of gut microbiota in intestinal inflammation with respect to diet and extrinsic stressors. *Microorganisms*, Vol. 7. https://doi.org/10.3390/microorganisms7080271

[11] Plunkett, C. H., & Nagler, C. R. (2017). The Influence of the Microbiome on Allergic Sensitization to Food. *The Journal of Immunology*, *198*(2), 581–589. https://doi.org/10.4049/jimmunol.1601266

[12] Lee, Byun, & Kim. (2019). Potential Role of the Microbiome in Acne: A Comprehensive Review. *Journal of Clinical Medicine*, *8*(7), 987. https://doi.org/10.3390/jcm8070987/

[13] Vighi, G., Marcucci, F., Sensi, L., Di Cara, G., & Frati, F. (2008, September). Allergy and the gastrointestinal system. *Clinical and Experimental Immunology*, Vol. 153, pp. 3–6. https://doi.org/10.1111/j.1365-

2249.2008.03713.x

[14] Schrom, K. P., Ahsanuddin, S., Baechtold, M., Tripathi, R., Ramser, A., & Baron, E. (2019). Acne Severity and Sleep Quality in Adults. *Clocks & Sleep*, *1*(4), 510–516. https://doi.org/10.3390/clockssleep1040039

[15] Mullington, J. M., Simpson, N. S., Meier-Ewert, H. K., & Haack, M. (2010, October). Sleep loss and inflammation. *Best Practice and Research: Clinical Endocrinology and Metabolism*, Vol. 24, pp. 775–784. https://doi.org/10.1016/j.beem.2010.08.014

[16] Almendros, I., & García-Río, F. (2017, April 1). Sleep apnoea, insulin resistance and diabetes: The first step is in the fat. *European Respiratory Journal*, Vol. 49. https://doi.org/10.1183/13993003.00179-2017

[17] Smith, R. P., Easson, C., Lyle, S. M., Kapoor, R., Donnelly, C. P., Davidson, E. J., ... Tartar, J. L. (2019). Gut microbiome diversity is associated with sleep physiology in humans. *PLoS ONE*, *14*(10). https://doi.org/10.1371/journal.pone.0222394/

[18] Valacchi, G., Rimbach, G., Saliou, C., Weber, S. U., & Packer, L. (2001). Effect of benzoyl peroxide on antioxidant status, NF-κB activity and interleukin-1α gene expression in human keratinocytes. *Toxicology*, *165*(2–3), 225–234. https://doi.org/10.1016/S0300-483X(01)00430-9

[19] Bowe, W. P., & Logan, A. C. (2010). Clinical implications of lipid peroxidation in acne vulgaris: Old wine in new bottles. *Lipids in Health and Disease*, *9*, 141. https://doi.org/10.1186/1476-511X-9-141

[20] Pullar, J. M., Carr, A. C., & Vissers, M. C. M. (2017, August 12). The roles of vitamin C in skin health. *Nutrients*, Vol. 9.

https://doi.org/10.3390/nu9080866

[21] Lobo, V., Patil, A., Phatak, A., & Chandra, N. (2010, July). Free radicals, antioxidants and functional foods: Impact on human health. *Pharmacognosy Reviews*, Vol. 4, pp. 118–126. https://doi.org/10.4103/0973-7847.70902

[22] Mills, O. H., Criscito, M. C., Schlesinger, T. E., Verdicchio, R., & Szoke, E. (2016). Addressing free radical oxidation in acne vulgaris. *Journal of Clinical and Aesthetic Dermatology*, *9*(1), 25–30. Retrieved from /pmc/articles/PMC4756869/?report=abstract

[23] Hazlewood, C., & Davies, M. J. (1996). Benzoyl peroxide-induced damage to DNA and its components: Direct evidence for the generation of base adducts, sugar radicals, and strand breaks. *Archives of Biochemistry and Biophysics*, *332*(1), 79–91. https://doi.org/10.1006/abbi.1996.0319

[24] Lundin, Knut & Alaedini, Armin. (2012). Non-celiac Gluten Sensitivity. Gastrointestinal endoscopy clinics of North America. 22. 723-34. 10.1016/j.giec.2012.07.006.

[25] Lönnerdal, B. (2000, May 01). Dietary factors influencing zinc absorption. Retrieved February 20, 2021, from https://doi.org/10.1093/jn/130.5.1378S

[26] Mercola, J. (2019, November 10). The Damaging Effects of Oxalates on the Human Body. Retrieved February 2, 2021, from Mercola website: https://articles.mercola.com/sites/articles/archive/2019/11/10/oxalic-toxicity.aspx

[27] Lajolo, F. M., & Genovese, M. I. (2002). Nutritional significance of lectins and enzyme inhibitors from legumes. *Journal of Agricultural and Food Chemistry*, *50*(22), 6592–6598. https://doi.org/10.1021/jf020191k

[28] Part 1: Soaking – Nuts. (n.d.). Retrieved February 2, 2021, from Jack Norris RD Blog website: https://jacknorrisrd.com/part-1-soaking-nuts/

[29] Kurzer, M. S. (2002). Hormonal effects of soy in premenopausal women and men. *Journal of Nutrition*, *132*(3). https://doi.org/10.1093/jn/132.3.570s

[30] Definition & Facts for Lactose Intolerance. (n.d.). Retrieved February 2, 2021, from National Institute of Diabetes and Digestive and Kidney Diseases (NIDDK) website: https://www.niddk.nih.gov/health-information/digestive-diseases/lactose-intolerance/definition-facts

[31] Stettler, N., Murphy, M. M., Barraj, L. M., Smith, K. M., & Ahima, R. S. (2013). Systematic review of clinical studies related to pork intake and metabolic syndrome or its components. *Diabetes, Metabolic Syndrome and Obesity: Targets and Therapy*, *6*, 347–357. https://doi.org/10.2147/DMSO.S51440

[32] Pappas, A. (2009). The relationship of diet and acne. *Dermato-Endocrinology*, *1*(5), 262–267. https://doi.org/10.4161/derm.1.5.10192

[33] Zinder, R., Cooley, R., Vlad, L. G., & Molnar, J. A. (2019, December 1). Vitamin A and Wound Healing. *Nutrition in Clinical Practice*, Vol. 34, pp. 839–849. https://doi.org/10.1002/ncp.10420

[34] Schagen, S. K., Zampeli, V. A., Makrantonaki, E., & Zouboulis, C. C. (2012, July). Discovering the link between nutrition and skin aging. *Dermato-Endocrinology*, Vol. 4, p. 298. https://doi.org/10.4161/derm.22876

[35] Reifen R. (2002). Vitamin A as an anti-inflammatory agent. *The Proceedings of the Nutrition Society*, *61*(3), 397–400.

https://doi.org/10.1079/PNS2002172

[36] Oba, K., & Kimura, S. (1980). Effects of vitamin A deficiency on thyroid function and serum thyroxine levels in the rat. *Journal of Nutritional Science and Vitaminology*, *26*(4), 327–334. https://doi.org/10.3177/jnsv.26.327

[37] Brown, M. J., Ferruzzi, M. G., Nguyen, M. L., Cooper, D. A., Eldridge, A. L., Schwartz, S. J., & White, W. S. (2004). Carotenoid bioavailability is higher from salads ingested with full-fat than with fat-reduced salad dressings as measured with electrochemical detection. *The American Journal of Clinical Nutrition*, *80*(2), 396–403. https://doi.org/10.1093/ajcn/80.2.396

[38] Fabbri, A. D. T., & Crosby, G. A. (2016, April 1). A review of the impact of preparation and cooking on the nutritional quality of vegetables and legumes. *International Journal of Gastronomy and Food Science*, Vol. 3, pp. 2–11. https://doi.org/10.1016/j.ijgfs.2015.11.001

[39] New market for tilapia. (2017, July 10). Retrieved February 2, 2021, from Food and Agriculture Organization of the United Nations website: http://www.fao.org/in-action/globefish/market-reports/resource-detail/en/c/989532/

[40] Alam, M. M., & Haque, M. M. (2021). Presence of Antibacterial Substances, Nitrofuran Metabolites and other Chemicals in Farmed Pangasius and Tilapia in Bangladesh: Probabilistic Health Risk Assessment. *Toxicology Reports*, *8*, 248–257. https://doi.org/10.1016/j.toxrep.2021.01.007

[41] Ribaya-Mercado, J. D. (2002). Influence of dietary fat on β-carotene absorption and bioconversion into vitamin A. *Nutrition Reviews*, *60*(4), 104–110. https://doi.org/10.1301/00296640260085831

[42] Stewart, T. J., & Bazergy, C. (2017). Thyroid autoimmunity in female post-adolescent acne: A case-control study. *Dermato-Endocrinology*, *9*(1), e1405198. https://doi.org/10.1080/19381980.2017.1405198

[43] Steptoe, A., Gibson, E. L., Vounonvirta, R., Williams, E. D., Hamer, M., Rycroft, J. A., ... Wardle, J. (2007). The effects of tea on psychophysiological stress responsivity and post-stress recovery: A randomised double-blind trial. *Psychopharmacology*, *190*(1), 81–89. https://doi.org/10.1007/s00213-006-0573-2

[44] Lane, J. D., Adcock, R. A., Williams, R. B., & Kuhn, C. M. (1990). Caffeine effects on cardiovascular and neuroendocrine responses to acute psychosocial stress and their relationship to level of habitual caffeine consumption. *Psychosomatic Medicine*, *52*(3), 320–336. https://doi.org/10.1097/00006842-199005000-00006

[45] Vongraviopap, S., & Asawanonda, P. (2016). Dark chocolate exacerbates acne. *International Journal of Dermatology*, *55*(5), 587–591. https://doi.org/10.1111/ijd.13188

[46] Gonzalez, C., Najera, O., Cortes, E., Toledo, G., Lopez, L., Betancourt, M., & Ortiz, R. (2002). Effects of fasting and intermittent fasting on rat hepatocarcinogenesis induced by diethylnitrosamine. *Teratogenesis Carcinogenesis and Mutagenesis*, *22*(2), 129–138. https://doi.org/10.1002/tcm.10005

[47] Kojima, N., & Shirao, T. (2007). Synaptic dysfunction and disruption of postsynaptic drebrin-actin complex: A study of neurological disorders accompanied by cognitive deficits. *Neuroscience Research*, *58*(1), 1–5. https://doi.org/10.1016/j.neures.2007.02.003

[48] Collier R. (2013). Intermittent fasting: the next big weight loss fad. CMAJ :

Canadian Medical Association journal = journal de l'Association medicale canadienne, 185(8), E321–E322. https://doi.org/10.1503/cmaj.109-4437

[49] Barnosky, A., Hoddy, K., Unterman, T., & Varady, K. (2014, June 12). Intermittent fasting vs daily calorie restriction for type 2 DIABETES prevention: A review of human findings. Retrieved February 04, 2021, from https://www.sciencedirect.com/science/article/abs/pii/S193152441400200X

[50] Martin, B., Mattson, M. P., & Maudsley, S. (2006). Caloric restriction and intermittent fasting: two potential diets for successful brain aging. Ageing research reviews, 5(3), 332–353. https://doi.org/10.1016/j.arr.2006.04.002

[51] Aly S. M. (2014). Role of intermittent fasting on improving health and reducing diseases. International journal of health sciences, 8(3), V–VI. https://doi.org/10.12816/0023985

[52] Godínez-Victoria, M., Campos-Rodriguez, R., Rivera-Aguilar, V., Lara-Padilla, E., Pacheco-Yepez, J., Jarillo-Luna, R. A., & Drago-Serrano, M. E. (2014). Intermittent fasting promotes bacterial clearance and intestinal IgA production in Salmonella typhimurium-infected mice. Scandinavian journal of immunology, 79(5), 315–324. https://doi.org/10.1111/sji.12163

[53] De Toledo, F. W., Grundler, F., Bergouignan, A., Drinda, S., & Michalsen, A. (2019). Safety, health improvement and well-being during a 4 to 21-day fasting period in an observational study including 1422 subjects. *PLoS ONE, 14*(1). https://doi.org/10.1371/journal.pone.0209353

[54] Choi, I. Y., Lee, C., & Longo, V. D. (2017). Nutrition and fasting mimicking diets in the prevention and treatment of autoimmune diseases and immunosenescence. *Molecular and Cellular Endocrinology, 455*, 4–12. https://doi.org/10.1016/j.mce.2017.01.042

[55] Longo, V. (n.d.). *The Longevity Diet: Discover the New Science Behind Stem Cell Activation and Regeneration to Slow Aging, Fight Disease, and Optimize Weight*. Retrieved February 2, 2021, from Health, Fitness & Dieting Kindle eBooks @ Amazon.com. website: https://www.amazon.com/dp/B073YMYX7H/ref=dp-kindle-redirect?_encoding=UTF8&btkr=1

[56] Prasanth, M. I., Sivamaruthi, B. S., Chaiyasut, C., & Tencomnao, T. (2019, February 1). A review of the role of green tea (camellia sinensis) in antiphotoaging, stress resistance, neuroprotection, and autophagy. *Nutrients*, Vol. 11, p. 474. https://doi.org/10.3390/nu11020474

[57] Diet soda and diabetes: Research and considerations. (n.d.). Retrieved February 2, 2021, from medical news today website: https://www.medicalnewstoday.com/articles/310909#diet-soda-and-diabetes

[58] Asghari, G., Farhadnejad, H., Teymoori, F., Mirmiran, P., Tohidi, M., & Azizi, F. (2018). High dietary intake of branched-chain amino acids is associated with an increased risk of insulin resistance in adults. *Journal of Diabetes*, *10*(5), 357–364. https://doi.org/10.1111/1753-0407.12639

[59] Rhonda, P. (Ph. D). (2019). *Fasting Q&A with Dr. Rhonda Patrick and Mike Maser*. https://www.foundmyfitness.com/episodes/zero-fasting-qa.

[60] Hodgson, A. B., Randell, R. K., & Jeukendrup, A. E. (2013, March). The effect of green tea extract on fat oxidation at rest and during exercise: Evidence of efficacy and proposed mechanisms. *Advances in Nutrition*, Vol. 4, pp. 129–140. https://doi.org/10.3945/an.112.003269

[61] Tang, G. (2010, May 1). Bioconversion of dietary provitamin A carotenoids to

vitamin A in humans. *American Journal of Clinical Nutrition*, Vol. 91, p. 1468S. https://doi.org/10.3945/ajcn.2010.28674G

[62] Naeem, Z. (2010). Vitamin d deficiency- an ignored epidemic. *International Journal of Health Sciences*, *4*(1), V–VI. Retrieved from http://www.ncbi.nlm.nih.gov/pubmed/21475519

[63] Yildizgören, M. T., & Togral, A. K. (2014). Preliminary evidence for vitamin D deficiency in nodulocystic acne. *Dermato-Endocrinology*, *6*(1). https://doi.org/10.4161/derm.29799

[64] Dreno, B., Moyse, D., Alirezai, M., Amblard, P., Auffret, N., Beylot, C., Poli, F. (2001). Multicenter Randomized Comparative Double-Blind Controlled Clinical Trial of the Safety and Efficacy of Zinc Gluconate versus Minocycline Hydrochloride in the Treatment of Inflammatory Acne vulgaris. *Dermatology*, *203*(2), 135–140. https://doi.org/10.1159/000051728

[65] Michaëlsson, G., Juhlin, L., & Vahlquist, A. (1977). Effects of Oral Zinc and Vitamin A in Acne. *Archives of Dermatology*, *113*(1), 31–36. https://doi.org/10.1001/archderm.1977.01640010033003

[66] Prasad, A. S. (2013, March). Discovery of human zinc deficiency: Its impact on human health and disease. *Advances in Nutrition*, Vol. 4, pp. 176–190. https://doi.org/10.3945/an.112.003210

[67] Ford, E. S., & Mokdad, A. H. (2003). Dietary magnesium intake in a national sample of U.S. adults. *Journal of Nutrition*, *133*(9), 2879–2882. https://doi.org/10.1093/jn/133.9.2879

[68] Kober, M. M., & Bowe, W. P. (2015, June 1). The effect of probiotics on

immune regulation, acne, and photoaging. *International Journal of Women's Dermatology*, Vol. 1, pp. 85–89. https://doi.org/10.1016/j.ijwd.2015.02.001

[69] Bowe, W. P., & Logan, A. C. (2011). Acne vulgaris, probiotics and the gut-brain-skin axis - Back to the future? *Gut Pathogens*, Vol. 3, p. 1. https://doi.org/10.1186/1757-4749-3-1

[70] Kang, B. S., Seo, J. G., Lee, G. S., Kim, J. H., Kim, S. Y., Han, Y. W., … Park, Y. M. (2009). Antimicrobial activity of enterocins from Enterococcus faecalis SL-5 against Propionibacterium acnes, the causative agent in acne vulgaris, and its therapeutic effect. *Journal of Microbiology*, *47*(1), 101–109. https://doi.org/10.1007/s12275-008-0179-y

[71] Dwyer, A. (2020, June 10). Probiotics for Acne & Skin Health. Retrieved February 2, 2021, from Probiotics Learning Lab website: https://www.optibacprobiotics.com/learning-lab/in-depth/general-health/can-probiotics-improve-skin-health.

[72] Wong, C. B., Odamaki, T., & Xiao, J. zhong. (2019, March 1). Beneficial effects of Bifidobacterium longum subsp. longum BB536 on human health: Modulation of gut microbiome as the principal action. *Journal of Functional Foods*, Vol. 54, pp. 506–519. https://doi.org/10.1016/j.jff.2019.02.002

[73] Bollinger, L., & LaFontaine, T. (2011). Exercise Programming for Insulin Resistance. *Strength and Conditioning Journal*, *33*(5), 44–47. https://doi.org/10.1519/SSC.0b013e31822599fb

[74] Michelle Brubaker. (2017, January 12). Exercise … it Does a Body Good: 20 Minutes Can Act as Anti-Inflammatory. Retrieved February 2, 2021, from UC San Diego Health website:

https://health.ucsd.edu/news/releases/pages/2017-01-12-exercise-can-act-as-anti-inflammatory.aspx.

[75] Monda, V., Villano, I., Messina, A., Valenzano, A., Esposito, T., Moscatelli, F., ... Messina, G. (2017, March 5). Exercise modifies the gut microbiota with positive health effects. *Oxidative Medicine and Cellular Longevity*, Vol. 2017. https://doi.org/10.1155/2017/3831972

[76] Exercising for Better Sleep . (n.d.). Retrieved February 2, 2021, from Johns Hopkins Medicine website: https://www.hopkinsmedicine.org/health/wellness-and-prevention/exercising-for-better-sleep

[77] Chaput, J. P., Carson, V., Gray, C. E., & Tremblay, M. S. (2014). Importance of all movement behaviors in a 24 hour period for overall health. *International Journal of Environmental Research and Public Health*, *11*(12), 12575–12581. https://doi.org/10.3390/ijerph111212575

[78] Liu YZ, Wang YX, Jiang CL. Inflammation: The Common Pathway of Stress-Related Diseases. *Front Hum Neurosci*. 2017;11:316. Published 2017 Jun 20. doi:10.3389/fnhum.2017.00316

[79] Foster, J. A., Rinaman, L., & Cryan, J. F. (2017, December 1). Stress & the gut-brain axis: Regulation by the microbiome. *Neurobiology of Stress*, Vol. 7, pp. 124–136. https://doi.org/10.1016/j.ynstr.2017.03.001

[80] Mullington, J. M., Simpson, N. S., Meier-Ewert, H. K., & Haack, M. (2010, October). Sleep loss and inflammation. *Best Practice and Research: Clinical Endocrinology and Metabolism*, Vol. 24, pp. 775–784. https://doi.org/10.1016/j.beem.2010.08.014

[81] Mesarwi, O., Polak, J., Jun, J., & Polotsky, V. Y. (2013, September). Sleep

Disorders and the Development of Insulin Resistance and Obesity. *Endocrinology and Metabolism Clinics of North America*, Vol. 42, pp. 617–634. https://doi.org/10.1016/j.ecl.2013.05.001

[82] Li, Y., Hao, Y., Fan, F., & Zhang, B. (2018). The Role of Microbiome in Insomnia, Circadian Disturbance and Depression. *Frontiers in Psychiatry*, 9, 669. https://doi.org/10.3389/fpsyt.2018.00669

[83] Saunders, M. A. (1976). Fluoride Toothpastes as a Cause of Acne-like Eruptions-Reply. *Archives of Dermatology*, *112*(7), 1033. https://doi.org/10.1001/archderm.1976.01630310079027

[84] KheradPisheh, Z., Mirzaei, M., Mahvi, A. H., Mokhtari, M., Azizi, R., Fallahzadeh, H., & Ehrampoush, M. H. (2018). Impact of drinking water fluoride on human thyroid hormones: A case-control study. *Scientific Reports*, *8*(1), 2674. https://doi.org/10.1038/s41598-018-20696-4

[85] Mead, M. N. (2008). Benefits of sunlight: a bright spot for human health. *Environmental Health Perspectives*, Vol. 116, p. A160. https://doi.org/10.1289/ehp.116-a160

[86] The Top 6 Raw Honey Benefits: Fights Infection, Heals Wounds, and More. (2019, November 15). Retrieved February 2, 2021, from Healthline website: https://www.healthline.com/health/food-nutrition/top-raw-honey-benefits

[87] New CDC report: More than 100 million Americans have diabetes or prediabetes |. (2017, July 18). Retrieved February 2, 2021, from CDC Online Newsroom website: https://www.cdc.gov/media/releases/2017/p0718-diabetes-report.html

[88] Boden, G., Sargrad, K., Homko, C., Mozzoli, M., & Stein, T. P. (2005). Effect of a low-carbohydrate diet on appetite, blood glucose levels, and insulin resistance in obese patients with type 2 diabetes.`

[89] Gu, Y., Zhao, A., Huang, F., Zhang, Y., Liu, J., Wang, C., ... Jia, W. (2013). Very low carbohydrate diet significantly alters the serum metabolic profiles in obese subjects. *Journal of Proteome Research*, *12*(12), 5801–5811. https://doi.org/10.1021/pr4008199

[90] Yuasa, M., Matsui, T., Ando, S., Ishii, Y., Sawamura, H., Ebara, S., & Watanabe, T. (2013). Consumption of a low-carbohydrate and high-fat diet (the ketogenic diet) exaggerates biotin deficiency in mice. Nutrition (Burbank, Los Angeles County, Calif.), 29(10), 1266–1270. https://doi.org/10.1016/j.nut.2013.04.011

[91] Mahabadi, N. (2020, July 21). Riboflavin deficiency. Retrieved February 18, 2021, from https://www.ncbi.nlm.nih.gov/books/NBK470460.

[92] Gray, N. A., Dhana, A., Stein, D. J., & Khumalo, N. P. (2019). Zinc and atopic dermatitis: a systematic review and meta-analysis. Journal of the European Academy of Dermatology and Venereology : JEADV, 33(6), 1042–1050. https://doi.org/10.1111/jdv.15524

[93] Dreno, B., Moyse, D., Alirezai, M., Amblard, P., Auffret, N., Beylot, C., ... Poli, F. (2001). Multicenter Randomized Comparative Double-Blind Controlled Clinical Trial of the Safety and Efficacy of Zinc Gluconate versus Minocycline Hydrochloride in the Treatment of Inflammatory Acne vulgaris. *Dermatology*, *203*(2), 135–140. https://doi.org/10.1159/000051728

[94] https://www.ncbi.nlm.nih.gov/pubmed/21521376

[95] Mancini, A., Di Segni, C., Raimondo, S., Olivieri, G., Silvestrini, A., Meucci, E., & Currò, D. (2016). Thyroid Hormones, Oxidative Stress, and

Inflammation. *Mediators of Inflammation*, Vol. 2016. https://doi.org/10.1155/2016/6757154

[96] Amino, N. (1988). 4 Autoimmunity and hypothyroidism. *Bailliere's Clinical Endocrinology and Metabolism*, 2(3), 591–617. https://doi.org/10.1016/S0950-351X(88)80055-7

[97] Kim, Y. A., & Park, Y. J. (2014). Prevalence and risk factors of subclinical thyroid disease. *Endocrinology and Metabolism*, Vol. 29, pp. 20–29. https://doi.org/10.3803/EnM.2014.29.1.20

[98] Cui, Y. Q., Jia, Y. J., Zhang, T., Zhang, Q. Bin, & Wang, X. M. (2012). Fucoidan protects against lipopolysaccharide-induced rat neuronal damage and inhibits the production of proinflammatory mediators in primary microglia. *CNS Neuroscience and Therapeutics*, 18(10), 827–833. https://doi.org/10.1111/j.1755-5949.2012.00372.x

[99] Kim, M. S., Kim, J. Y., Choi, W. H., & Lee, S. S. (2008). Effects of seaweed supplementation on blood glucose concentration, lipid profile, and antioxidant enzyme activities in patients with type 2 diabetes mellitus. *Nutrition Research and Practice*, 2(2), 62. https://doi.org/10.4162/nrp.2008.2.2.62

[100] Marudhupandi, T., Ajith Kumar, T. T., Lakshmana Senthil, S., & Nanthini Devi, K. (2014). In vitro antioxidant properties of fucoidan fractions from Sargassum tenerrimum. *Pakistan Journal of Biological Sciences*, 17(3), 402–407. https://doi.org/10.3923/pjbs.2014.402.407

[101] Ullrich, I. H., Peters, P. J., & Albrink, M. J. (1982). Effect of low—carbohydrate diets high in either fat or protein on thyroid function, plasma insulin, glucose, and triglycerides in healthy young adults. *Journal of the American College of Nutrition*, 4(4), 451–459.

https://doi.org/10.1080/07315724.1985.10720087

[102] Betsy, A., Binitha, M. P., & Sarita, S. (2013). Zinc deficiency associated with hypothyroidism: An overlooked cause of severe alopecia. *International Journal of Trichology*, *5*(1), 40–42. https://doi.org/10.4103/0974-7753.114714

[103] Mackawy, A. M. H., Al-Ayed, B. M., & Al-Rashidi, B. M. (2013). Vitamin D Deficiency and Its Association with Thyroid Disease. *International Journal of Health Sciences*, *7*(3), 267–275. https://doi.org/10.12816/0006054

Made in the USA
Las Vegas, NV
04 March 2025